Natural Products and Therapeutics

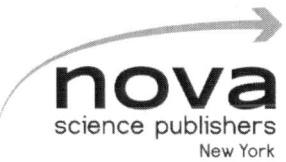

Natural Products and Therapeutics

Ginger's Antimicrobial, Anti-Nausea and Anti-Osteoarthritic Activities
Diana R. Cundell, PhD (Editor)
2021. ISBN: 978-1-68507-117-2 (Hardcover)
2021. ISBN: 978-1-68507-165-3 (eBook)

The Bible and Medicinal Plants: The Healing Power of Natural Medicines
Mohamad Hesam Shahrajabian
Ted Trandahl
2021. ISBN: 978-1-53619-391-6 (Hardcover)
2021. ISBN: 978-1-53619-431-9 (eBook)

Basil, Chinese Onion, Pyrethrum, Shallot and Tremella: Powerful Medicinal Plants to Live an Organic Lifestyle
Mohamad Hesam Shahrajabian, Ph.D.
Diorge Jonatas Marmitt, Ph.D.
Wenli Sun, Ph.D.
Qi Cheng, Ph.D.
2021. ISBN: 978-1-53619-425-8 (eBook)

Ginkgo biloba, Leek, Peganum harmala, and Smilax china: Power of Medicinal Plants for Organic Life
Wenli Sun, PhD
Mohamad Hesam Shahrajabian, PhD
Qi Cheng, PhD
2021. ISBN: 978-1-53619-271-1 (eBook)

Curcuma longa and Its Health Effects. Volume 2
Noboru Motohashi, PhD (Editor)
2020. ISBN: 978-1-53618-088-6 (Hardcover)
2020. ISBN: 978-1-53618-089-3 (eBook)

More information about this series can be found at
https://novapublishers.com/product-category/series/natural-products-and-therapeutics/

Isla Kermode
Editor

Ginger and its Health Benefits

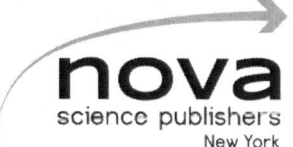

Copyright © 2022 by Nova Science Publishers, Inc.

All rights reserved. No part of this book may be reproduced, stored in a retrieval system or transmitted in any form or by any means: electronic, electrostatic, magnetic, tape, mechanical photocopying, recording or otherwise without the written permission of the Publisher.

We have partnered with Copyright Clearance Center to make it easy for you to obtain permissions to reuse content from this publication. Simply navigate to this publication's page on Nova's website and locate the "Get Permission" button below the title description. This button is linked directly to the title's permission page on copyright.com. Alternatively, you can visit copyright.com and search by title, ISBN, or ISSN.

For further questions about using the service on copyright.com, please contact:
Copyright Clearance Center
Phone: +1-(978) 750-8400   Fax: +1-(978) 750-4470   E-mail: info@copyright.com.

NOTICE TO THE READER

The Publisher has taken reasonable care in the preparation of this book, but makes no expressed or implied warranty of any kind and assumes no responsibility for any errors or omissions. No liability is assumed for incidental or consequential damages in connection with or arising out of information contained in this book. The Publisher shall not be liable for any special, consequential, or exemplary damages resulting, in whole or in part, from the readers' use of, or reliance upon, this material. Any parts of this book based on government reports are so indicated and copyright is claimed for those parts to the extent applicable to compilations of such works.

Independent verification should be sought for any data, advice or recommendations contained in this book. In addition, no responsibility is assumed by the Publisher for any injury and/or damage to persons or property arising from any methods, products, instructions, ideas or otherwise contained in this publication.

This publication is designed to provide accurate and authoritative information with regard to the subject matter covered herein. It is sold with the clear understanding that the Publisher is not engaged in rendering legal or any other professional services. If legal or any other expert assistance is required, the services of a competent person should be sought. FROM A DECLARATION OF PARTICIPANTS JOINTLY ADOPTED BY A COMMITTEE OF THE AMERICAN BAR ASSOCIATION AND A COMMITTEE OF PUBLISHERS.

Additional color graphics may be available in the e-book version of this book.

Library of Congress Cataloging-in-Publication Data

ISBN: 978-1-68507-695-5

Published by Nova Science Publishers, Inc. † New York

Contents

Preface		vii
Chapter 1	**Health Benefits of Ginger in Gastrointestinal Disorders**	1
	Hatice Gül Anlar	
Chapter 2	**Potential Benefits of Ginger in Maintenance of Oral Health**	19
	C. Pushpalatha, Kavita Kamondur and Arshiya Shakir	
Chapter 3	**Image Processing of Ginger Extract via Microwave- Assisted Hydrodistillation**	37
	Siti Nuurul Huda Mohammad Azmin and Mohd Shukri Mat Nor	
Chapter 4	**Effects of Ginger (*Zingiber officinale* Roscoe 1807) on Health Promotion**	55
	Karina Zanoti Fonseca, Ferlando Lima Santos and Franceli da Silva	
Bibliography		65
Index		137

Preface

Ginger is a flowering plant originally from Southeast Asia that is commonly used as a spice and is well-known for its various health benefits. Several of these benefits are described in detail in the four chapters of this book. Chapter One provides knowledge about ginger's beneficial effects in the treatment of gastrointestinal disorders. Chapter Two highlights the composition and properties of ginger, oral application, and its future scope in dentistry. Chapter Three includes a case study of ginger extraction using microwave-assisted hydrodistillation to compare images from before and after the extraction process of ginger. Lastly, Chapter Four addresses the state of the art of research on the use of ginger in health promotion.

Chapter 1 - Gastrointestinal (GI) disorders are the term used to refer to any condition or disease that occurs within the gastrointestinal tract. These disorders affect a lot of people and decreased their life quality. Ginger (Zingiber officinale) has been used in the kitchen as a spice for centuries. Promising data from epidemiological as well as in vitro and animal studies have claimed that consumption of ginger may be useful in the treatment and also prevention of GI diseases such as nausea and vomiting, irritable bowel syndrome, Helicobacter pylori infection, and gastric ulcerations. This chapter aims to provide knowledge about the general information about ginger and its beneficial health effects on GI diseases.

Chapter 2 - Ginger rhizomes or Zingiberofficinale is a perennial crop grown in tropical and subtropical regions worldwide. It has been used as traditional medicine for 2500 years to alleviate headaches, cold and gastrointestinal disorders. It is also used as an alternative medicine to treat rheumatological, musculoskeletal, and dyslipidemia conditions [1]. Minerals, vitamins, and phytochemicals are abundant in ginger. Recently, ginger has received a lot of interest in dentistry to avoid tooth problems. Ginger has no toxicity hence it is regarded as safe (GRAS) by the US Food and Drug Administration [2]. The polyphenolic ketones or Gingerols present in ginger are mainly responsible for pharmacological effects such as antioxidant, anti-inflammatory, and antimicrobial activities. It was first reported in the early 1980s that Ginger has anti-inflammatory activity since it has the potential to inhibit prostaglandins synthesis. Gingerols and Shogaols present in Ginger exhibit pharmacological characteristics that are similar to dual-acting non-steroidal anti-inflammatory medications. The Ginger antioxidant activity is responsible for protection against radiation toxicity and lethality. Ginger exhibits antibacterial activity against Streptococcus mutans and Streptococcus sanguinis. Since ginger has a wide range of pharmacotherapeutic characteristics, it has been used to treat oral diseases [3-5]. This chapter highlights the composition and properties of ginger, oral application, and the future scope of ginger in dentistry.

Chapter 3 - Extraction techniques become the primary process to obtain a good quality of plant extraction yield. However, the extraction technique efficiency could be determined by comparing the image processing before and after the extraction process. Image processing of the extract is an important technique to determine the factors affecting the success of the extraction yield. Therefore, this chapter reviews the state-of-the-art development for plant processing and the fundamentals of microwave-assisted hydrodistillation extraction methods. The case study of ginger extraction using microwave-assisted hydrodistillation was demonstrated where the images before and after the extraction processes of ginger were revealed. This chapter also discusses the comparison of the morphological images of the ginger extract.

Chapter 4 - Ginger (Zingiber officinale Roscoe 1807) is a perennial monocot rhizome of the family Zingiberaceae native from south east Asia. It is widely used worldwide as spice and as beverage flavor, mainly in Asian products. Ginger is not only used as food, but also in the traditional Asian medicine. Several studies have focused on the health benefits of ginger consumption based on the fact that India and China have been traditionally using it to treat asthma, headache, infectious diseases, rheumatoid arthritis and helminthiasis. Its main effects are related to its anti-inflammatory, anti-tumor, anti-hyperglycemic and anti-lipidemic activities. One of its bioactive compounds, gingerol, prevents hyperlipidemia induced by lipid-rich diets by regulating the expression of enzymes involved in cholesterol homeostasis. Ginger is considered a safe and effective antidiabetic adjuvant and shows beneficial effects on lipid profile, insulin resistance and weight loss. Its protective effects against cancer are among its most studied properties and are related to the induction of tumor cell apoptosis and inhibition of cell proliferation. This chapter addresses the state of the art of research on the use of ginger in health promotion.

Chapter 1

Health Benefits of Ginger in Gastrointestinal Disorders

Hatice Gül Anlar[*]

Department of Pharmaceutical Toxicology, Faculty of Pharmacy, Zonguldak Bulent Ecevit University, Zonguldak, Turkey

Abstract

Gastrointestinal (GI) disorders are the term used to refer to any condition or disease that occurs within the gastrointestinal tract. These disorders affect a lot of people and decreased their life quality. Ginger (*Zingiber officinale*) has been used in the kitchen as a spice for centuries. Promising data from epidemiological as well as *in vitro* and animal studies have claimed that consumption of ginger may be useful in the treatment and also prevention of GI diseases such as nausea and vomiting, irritable bowel syndrome, *Helicobacter pylori* infection, and gastric ulcerations. This chapter aims to provide knowledge about the general information about ginger and its beneficial health effects on GI diseases.

Keywords: ginger, gastrointestinal disorders, health, *Zingiber officinale*

Introduction

Zingiber officinale also called ginger is a member of the Zingiberaceae family and is native to Asia but is now cultivated in the West Indies, Africa, India, and other tropical regions. Ginger spice is prepared from the underground stem (rhizome) of the plant and it comes in different colors from white to brown.

---

[*] Corresponding Author's Email: haticegulanlar@gmail.com.

In: Ginger and its Health Benefits
Editor: Isla Kermode
ISBN: 978-1-68507-695-5
© 2022 Nova Science Publishers, Inc.

This spice has been used in the kitchen since the 13th century with a great diversity of uses (Langner, Greifenberg, and Gruenwald 1998). It can be consumed in food additives, drinks, and food products like curry powder, confectionaries, soups, jams, and flour products (Singletary 2010). Besides, it has been used in folk medicine for the therapy of gastrointestinal disorders, arthritis, menstrual irregularities, asthma, and diabetes (Ali et al. 2008a). There is evidence that ginger has also ameliorative effects in nausea caused by pregnancy or other reasons, inflammation, cancer, diabetes, and high cholesterol (Grzanna, Lindmark, and Frondoza 2005, Afzal et al. 2001, Shukla and Singh 2007, Ghayur et al. 2005).

This chapter aims to provide information about the health benefits of ginger in gastrointestinal disorders. Also, general information, chemistry, safety, and bioavailability of ginger were provided.

Chemistry

Ginger includes various volatile and non-volatile compounds, and their concentration differs relating to growing situations, temperature, harvesting, and processing. Volatile compounds such as camphene, b-phellandrene, curcumin, cineole, geranyl acetate, terpineol, terpenes, borneol, geraniol, limonene, b-elemene, zingiberol, linalool, a-zingiberene, bsesquiphellandrene, b-bisabolene, zingiberenol, and a-farmesene created the characteristic essence of ginger (Chrubasik, Pittler, and D. Roufogalis 2005). The non-volatile compounds like the gingerolsshogaols, paradols, and zingerone provide pungency and warm pungent sense in the mouth (Govindarajan 1982).

Gingerols are a series of chemical homologs differentiated by the length of their unbranched alkyl chains which can be found in fresh ginger. [3–6]-, [8]-, [10]-, and [12]-gingerols and having a side-chain with 7–10, 12, 14, or 16 carbon atoms, respectively as the principal active ingredients. 6-gingerol is the most abundant of all the gingerols (Yoshikawa et al. 1993).

Gingerols are thermolabile and they change shogaols rapidly via dehydration. And shogaols can convert to paradols via hydrogenation. Neral, capsaicin, gingediol, galanolactone, gingesulfonic acid, galactosylglycerols, gingerglycolipids, diarylheptanoids, and phytosterols are other constituents of ginger (Haniadka et al. 2013, Ali et al. 2008b).

Safety

Ginger has been classified as generally recognized as safe (GRAS) by the Food and Drug Administration (FDA) (Moneret-Vautrin et al. 2002).

In the animal study, ginger powder at the doses of 500, 1000, and 2000 mg/kg body weight was given to male and female rats for 35 days by gavage. Results of this study showed no relation between ginger and mortality, abnormal conditions in the behavior, growth or food intake, or hematological and biochemical parameters (Rong et al. 2009).

Also in human studies with ginger, only a few adverse reactions such as mild gastrointestinal distress, heartburn, oral irritation, and diarrhea have been reported. It can be demonstrated that that ginger at the higher dose of 2 g/d resulted in minor toxic effects in humans (Chrubasik, Pittler, and Roufogalis 2005).

Bioavailability

There is restricted information about the bioavailability of the ginger components. When 3 mg/kg ginger was given to rats intravenously, it is rapidly eliminated from the blood with a half-life ($t_{1/2}$) of 7.2 minutes due to the liver metabolism (Ali et al. 2008a).

Microsomal preparations were extracted from humans and rodents and used for the investigation of [6]-gingerol metabolization. It was shown that [6]-gingerol is metabolized to a mixed of glucuronidated polar metabolites (Pfeiffer et al. 2006, Surh and Lee 1994). Also, gut microorganisms can have a role in the metabolism of [6]-gingerol (Nakazawa and Ohsawa 2002).

After a healthy person took 100 mg to 2 g of ginger orally, gingerol and shogaol constituents were quickly absorbed and found in the serum especially as glucuronide conjugates, and there were no free forms. Therefore, nonconjugated ginger compounds can have limited clinical efficacy. Administration of 1.5 and 2 g dose of ginger can cause maximum serum concentrations of ginger metabolites (Zick et al. 2008).

Beneficial Effects on Gastrointestinal Disorders

The gastrointestinal system (GIS) is an important organ system that digests foods to extract, absorb food nutrients and eject the remaining waste as feces in humans and animals. The mouth, esophagus, stomach, and intestines are part of the GI tract which is under the control of the neurohormonal system. The stomach secretes proteolytic enzymes and strong acids to digest the food and after that, partly digested food send to the ileum for further digestion and absorption. Disorders such as dyspepsy, burping, bloat, gastroenteritis, and epigastric discomfort are moderate, but gastric ulcers and cancer cause severe morbidity and mortality. There are a lot of medicines that can be used for the treatment of GIS diseases but they have unwanted side effects, because of that people tend to use herbal medicine (Johnson et al. 1984).

Exercise-Induced Gastrointestinal Disturbances

Exercise-induced gastrointestinal disturbances affect people frequently and it causes mild stomach discomfort and even severe diarrhea, in the upper and lower of the gastrointestinal tract. It is more common with the consumption of beverages either before or during exercise. In a study conducted with recreational athletes (n = 40), beneficial activities of ginger juice on the frequency and severity of gastrointestinal disturbance during and after exercise were investigated. Each participant completed a 5 km run, after that upper and lower GI symptoms, before and after exercise were assessed by questionnaire. It has been shown that ginger administration decreased gastrointestinal problems after exercise (Ball, Ashley, and Stradling 2015).

Mode of Action

There are several mechanisms of action of ginger on gastrointestinal disorders. First is the free radical scavenging activity of ginger which is explained by reactive oxygen species (ROS) and reactive nitrogen species (RNS) play in the pathogenesis of a lot of diseases (Jagetia, Baliga, and Venkatesh 2004). Second, ginger and its constituents inhibit lipid peroxidation *in vitro* (Reddy and Lokesh 1992). Ginger also induces antioxidant defense systems which contained antioxidant molecules and enzymes (Shanmugam et al. 2010). Several studies have shown that ginger has anti-inflammatıry properties and modulate detoxifying enzymes (Haniadka et al. 2013).

Mechanism of gingers beneficial effects of dyspepsia was investigated by Ghayur M.N. and Gilani H. (Ghayur and Gilani 2005) in different animals such as rabbit, mice, and guinea pig. Their results showed that ginger has both spasmogenic and spasmolytic effects and is mediated through cholinergic and calcium antagonist mechanisms.

Gingers' anti-emetic effects are directly on the GI tract without central nervous system side effects (Micklefield et al. 1999). [6]-gingerol and 6-shogaol are the principal constituents that are responsible for the anti-nauseant effects of ginger and it increases intestinal motility and self-generated peristaltic activity. These effects decrease the gastrointestinal signals to central chemoreceptors which lead to reducing the emotion of nausea (Suekawa et al. 1984).

Nausea and Vomiting of Pregnancy

Nausea and/or vomiting of pregnancy (NVP) has been reported by approximately 50–90% of pregnant women especially in the first trimester of pregnancy but its cause is unknown (Lee and Saha 2011). NVP also is known as morning sickness, can range from a moderate feeling of seasickness to serious nausea and vomiting. When nausea and vomiting are too serious, it causes starvation and dehydration and treats the lives of the mother and her child. This condition is called "Hyperemesis gravidarum" which occurred in 1–2% of pregnant women (Quinla and Hill 2003).

Vitamin B6, ginger, and other herbal treatments such as peppermint and Cannabis have been used as an alternative treatment for NVP (Meltzer 2000). But only ginger was investigated in pregnant women by clinical trials. In the animal studies, there was no sign of teratogenicity associated with ginger (Weidner and Sigwart 2000, Wilkinson 2000). Also, Vutyavanich et al. (Vutyavanich, Kraisarin, and Ruangsri 2001) reported no adverse activities of ginger on the consequence of pregnancy.

Motherisk Program in Toronto, Canada showed that over 50% of the women consumed ginger tea or tablet (Hollyer et al. 2002). In the study of Smith et al. (Smith et al. 2004), ginger and vitamin B6 were compared and ginger decreased the symptoms of nausea as vitamin B6. Also, the risk of pregnancy loss was decreased in the ginger group compared to the vitamin B6 group. Portnoi et al. (Portnoi et al. 2003) showed that ginger has moderate effects on the treatment of NVP and it didn't induce major malformations.

Aikins (Aikins Murphy 1998) and Fischer-Rasmussen et al. (Fischer-Rasmussen et al. 1991) demonstrated that ginger may be useful as a safe and efficient antinauseant and they recommend 0.5 to 1.0 g of ginger per day for the alleviation of morning sickness. In the recent review of Bryer (Bryer 2005) it was reported that there is enough proof for the beneficial activity of ginger in the treatment of NVP. Also, a more recent systematic literature searches demonstrated that ginger has beneficial effects on the treatment for NVP in pregnancy (Borrelli et al. 2005).

Still, there are some concerns about ginger in the treatment of NVP. Ginger has thromboxane synthetase inhibitor effects and therefore, it may influence the testosterone-binding receptors in the fetus which lead to changes in the sex steroid-dependent differentiation of the fetal brain. Therefore, some researchers said that ginger should not be used in pregnant women until its testosterone binding effects clearly understand (Backon 1991). But further studies did not report any severe changes in thromboxane synthesis after two weeks of treatment of 40 g cooked ginger (Janssen et al. 1996, Lumb 1994). It can also inhibit platelet aggregation and induce the biosynthesis of prostacyclin (Srivastava 1986, Srivas 1984). Thus, the interaction between antiplatelet drugs and ginger should be considered.

Although it has been suggested that ginger has antiemetic properties, ginger has been clinically studied only in the NVP treatment (Chrubasik, Pittler, and Roufogalis 2005, Bone et al. 1990, Parveen et al. 2015). The Meta-analysis studies didn't confirm any antiemetic effects in the post-operative and in-motion sickness or nausea/vomiting relating to other reasons (Emma Westfall 2004).

Irritable Bowel Syndrome

Irritable Bowel Syndrome (IBS) is defined as abdomen pain and changes in intestinal habits which is a widespread chronic disease. The efficiency of medicine in the treatment of IBS is limited and therefore, approximately 40% of patients prefer alternative treatments (van Tilburg et al. 2008).

In a clinical study, 45 IBS patients have divided into there groups i.e., placebo, one gram, or two grams of ginger/day for 28 days. IBS Severity Scale (IBS-SS) was investigated with five factors including severity and frequency of pain, abdominal distension, bowel dissatisfaction, and interfering with life which was rated on a 0–100 scale. Adequate Relief Rating Scale (ARRS) was investigated with this question "In the last week, have you had enough relief of your abdominal pain and other symptoms of IBS (yes or no)?" As a result of this study, 57.1% of patients responded to placebo while 46.7% to 1 g and 33.3% to 2 g of ginger ($p > 0.05$). Even though patients weel tolerated ginger, it did not show a significant effect compared to placebo. But this study was conducted in a small group, further large trials are necessary to draw any definite outcome about the effectiveness of ginger in the treatment of IBS (van Tilburg et al. 2014).

Functional Abdominal Pain Disorders

Functional abdominal pain disorders (FAPDs) influence 10–25% of school-age children. It significantly decreased quality of life because it causes school absenteeism, sleeping disorders, comorbid somatic pains, depression, and anxiety (Varni et al. 2015, Carlson et al. 2014). The diagnosis of FAPDs was done according to the Rome IV criteria including irritable bowel syndrome (IBS), functional abdominal pain (FAP), functional dyspepsia (FD), and abdominal migraine (Edwards, Friesen, and Schurman 2018).

The biopsychosocial model showed that multiple factors such as visceral hypersensitivity, gut dysbiosis, motility abnormalities, abnormal gastrointestinal reactivity response to physiological (e.g., dietary), or other factors such as toxins or psychological stress can cause FAPDs (Beinvogl et al. 2018). Drug therapies in the treatment of FAPDs have some side effects (Chiou and Nurko 2011). As a result of this, complementary and traditional therapies draw attention from the parent of children with FAPDs (Pike et al. 2013).

Hu et al. (Hu et al. 2011) investigated the beneficial effects of ginger on gastric motility and emptying, abdominal symptoms, and hormones in 11 Chinese patients. Effects of ginger were compared to placebo after. One hour later, pain, nausea, abdominal discomfort, bloating and abdominal fullness, plasma glucagon-like peptide-1 (GLP-1), motilin, and ghrelin concentrations in the blood were analyzed. Ginger significantly decreased median gastric half-emptying time ($p < 0.05$). But it didn't affect nausea or abdominal discomfort. Since it was known that impaired gastric emptying can contribute to FAPDs (Di Stefano et al. 2005), ginger may be effective in the treatment of FAPDs. Similarly, Lazzini et al. (Lazzini et al. 2016) indicated that Prodigest which is a standardized extract of ginger and artichoke significantly stimulated gastric emptying in healthy people ($p < 0.001$).

A randomized controlled trial with fourteen healthy young male volunteers showed that after 1 gram-ginger consumption enhances the relaxivity of the lower esophageal sphincter, to decrease esophageal contraction velocity, and that these activities possibly mediate the anti-flatulent effects of ginger (Lohsiriwat et al. 2010).

The effects of Daikenchuto (DKT) which is mixed of Zingiberis rhizoma (processed ginger), Ginseng radix (*Panax ginseng*), and *Zanthoxyli fructus* (Japanese pepper) was assessed in 10 patients with chronic constipation and bloating and it remarkably ameliorated the quality of life of patients (Yuki et al. 2015).

Motion Sickness or Seasickness

It is not clear that ginger has beneficial effects on motion sickness or kinetosis (Cohen 2007). In the experimental and clinical studies, it was shown that ginger decreased symptoms relating to motion sickness in comparison with controls or antiemetic drugs but these effects were not statistically significant. It should be taken into consideration that in these studies, ginger doses, latency, and length of the response period monitored were highly different (Ernst and Pittler 2000). Also, the mechanism of decreasing motion sickness effects of ginger has not been well characterized. It was suggested that antiemetic effects of ginger for motion sickness are only effective in the GIS but not in the central nervous system (Lumb 1993).

Nausea Due to Chemotherapy/Radiotherapy

The beneficial effects of hydroalcoholic extract of ginger on the radiotherapy-induced nausea were investigated in rats and it was found that ginger blocked the saccharin avoidance response (Sharma et al. 2005, Haksar et al. 2006). Ginger also prevented emesis induced by cisplatin in healthy mongrel dogs. The ranging of effectiveness was granisetron>acetone extract > ethanolic extract (Sharma et al. 1997). In an animal study conducted in minks, the antiemetic activity of gingerol was compared to ondansetron, and gingerols effect was found to be similar to ondansetron (Qian et al. 2010). But there is not enough evidence in the animal studies about gingers antiemetic effects in reducing the adverse effects of chemotherapeutic agents (Frisch et al. 1995, Seynaeve, De Mulder, and Verweij 1991).

Results of human studies about the beneficial effects of ginger on nausea due to chemotherapy/radiotherapy are controversial (Manusirivithaya et al. 2004, Hickok et al. 2007). Ginger didn't decrease the prevalence or intention of acute or delayed chemotherapy-induced nausea and vomiting when given with HT3 receptor antagonists and/or aprepitant (Zick et al. 2009). Therefore, further studies are needed before recommendations can be made (Singletary 2010).

Postoperative Nausea and Vomiting

Results of human studies which analyzed ginger's ameliorative effects of nausea and vomiting after surgery are not consistent. There are some differences in dosages of ginger and timing of outcome measurements (Chaiyakunapruk et al. 2006, Thompson and Potter 2006, Tavlan et al. 2006). In those studies demonstrated the activity of ginger, generally, no adverse effects were reported (Singletary 2010).

Gastric Emptying

There is also evidences that ginger reversed cisplatin or pyrogallol-induced delay in gastric emptying time (Sharma and Gupta 1998, Gupta and Sharma 2001).

Gastric Ulcerations

It has been known that non-steroidal anti-inflammatory drugs cause gastric ulcers by producing free radicals, preventing prostaglandin synthesis, and stimulating acid secretion. In the preclinical studies, ginger (500 mg/kg) was given orally to rats and it ameliorated anti-ulcerogenic activity induced by indomethacin (al-Yahya et al. 1989). Also, ginger oil at doses of 0.5 and 1 g/kg has protective effects on ulcers induced by aspirin and pylorus ligation which is a common model of gastric ulceration in Wistar rats (Khushtar et al. 2009).

Ethanol also causes ulcers by producing free radicals. Acetone extract of ginger (1000 mg/kg), zingiberene (100 mg/kg), and 6-gingerol were given orally to rats and it significantly decreased gastric lesions induced by HCl/ethanol. Phytochemical components of ginger such as bsesquiphellandrene, b-bisabolene, ar-curcumin, and 6-shogaol have also gastroprotective activity against HCl/ethanol-induced gastric lesions (Yamahara et al. 1988).

It was shown that ginger increased the activities of antioxidant enzymes such as superoxide dismutase (SOD), catalase (CAT), glutathione peroxidase (GPx), and glutathione s transferase (GST) in rats (Prakash and Srinivasan 2010). Another study by Ko and Leung demonstrated ginger's gastroprotective effects on the acetic acid induced ulcer (Ko and Leung 2010).

Helicobacter Pylori (H. Pylori) Infection

Helicobacter pylori is a gram-negative, microaerophilic bacterium that is classified as a human carcinogen by the International Agency for Research on Cancer (IARC). It has been known to be a major reason for peptic ulcer and gastric cancer (IARC, 1994). Various extracts of ginger, the oil of ginger, and gingerol-containing fractions inhibited the growth of H. Pylori stains even if highly virulent CagA+ strains (Mahady et al. 2003).

Ginger-free phenolic and hydrolyzed phenolic fractions blocked H. pylori growth better than lansoprazole. It scavenged free radicals, protect DNA, and decreased lipid peroxidation (Siddaraju and Dharmesh 2007). Animal studies have also demonstrated that pretreatment with the standardized ginger extract (100 mg/kg) reduced H. pylori growth and also acute and chronic mucosal and submucosal inflammation, cryptitis, epithelial cell degeneration, and erosion caused by *H. Pylori* (Gaus et al. 2009).

Hyperglycemia-Induced Gastric Dysrhythmias

Gastropathy is one of the common diabetic complications that affect patient's life. The mechanism of diabetic gastropathy is complicated but motor disturbances such as delayed gastric emptying, decreased fundic tone, pylorospasm, and antral contractions are known to be major pathways. Hyperglycaemia can cause a delay in gastric emptying and gastric slow-wave dysrhythmias can occur in diabetic patients. In a clinical study with healthy volunteers, ginger reduced the induction of tachygastria in response to acute hyperglycemia when compared to a placebo. Besides, ginger did not affect the slow-wave disruptions caused by 400 mg of misoprostol. These results demonstrated that gingers antidysrhythmic effects occurred by its preventive effect on the production of prostaglandin during periods of hyperglycemia (Gonlachanvit et al. 2003).

Conclusion

Gastrointestinal diseases are affecting a significant proportion of the population worldwide. Ginger has been used as a food and spice for centuries. Recently its beneficial effects on gastrointestinal and inflammatory conditions draw attention. There is plenty of evidence that ginger may be safe and effective for NVP when used at recommended doses for short periods. Although there is no clinical support for its harmful effects, there is some safety concerns have been raised when pregnant women used ginger in large doses. Therefore, further epidemiological as well as *in vivo* and *in vitro* studies are required the confirm the useful effects of ginger on gastrointestinal disorders.

References

Afzal, M., Al-Hadidi, D., Menon, M., Pesek, J. & Dhami, M. S. (2001). "Ginger: an ethnomedical, chemical and pharmacological review." *Drug Metabol Drug Interact*, *18* (3-4), 159-90.

Aikins Murphy, P. (1998). "Alternative therapies for nausea and vomiting of pregnancy." *Obstet Gynecol*, *91* (1), 149-55.

al-Yahya, M. A., Rafatullah, S., Mossa, J. S., Ageel, A. M., Parmar, N. S. & Tariq, M. (1989). "Gastroprotective activity of ginger zingiber officinale rosc., in albino rats." *Am J Chin Med*, *17* (1-2), 51-6. doi: 10.1142/s0192415x89000097.

Ali, B. H., Blunden, G., Tanira, M. O. & Nemmar, A. (2008a). "Some phytochemical, pharmacological and toxicological properties of ginger (Zingiber officinale Roscoe): a review of recent research." *Food Chem Toxicol*, *46* (2), 409-20. doi: 10.1016/j.fct.2007.09.085.

Ali, Badreldin H., Gerald Blunden, Musbah O. Tanira. & Abderrahim Nemmar. (2008b). "Some phytochemical, pharmacological and toxicological properties of ginger (Zingiber officinale Roscoe): A review of recent research." *Food and Chemical Toxicology*, *46* (2), 409-420. doi: https://doi.org/10.1016/j.fct.2007.09.085.

Backon, J. (1991). "Ginger in preventing nausea and vomiting of pregnancy; a caveat due to its thromboxane synthetase activity and effect on testosterone binding." *Eur J Obstet Gynecol Reprod Biol*, *42* (2), 163-4.

Ball, Derek, Ashley, G. & Stradling, H. (2015). Exercise-induced gastrointestinal disturbances: potential amelioration with a ginger containing beverage, *Proceedings of The Nutrition Society*, *74*. DOI:10.1017/S0029665115002128.

Beinvogl, Beate, Elizabeth Burch, Julie Snyder, Neil Schechter, Amy Hale, Yoshiko Okazaki, Fiona Paul, Karen Warman. & Samuel Nurko. (2018). "Multidisciplinary Treatment of Pediatric Functional Gastrointestinal Disorders Results in Improved Pain

and Functioning." *Clinical gastroenterology and hepatology: the official clinical practice journal of the American Gastroenterological Association.*
Bone, M. E., Wilkinson, D. J., Young, J. R., McNeil, J. & Charlton, S. (1990). "Ginger root--a new antiemetic. The effect of ginger root on postoperative nausea and vomiting after major gynaecological surgery." *Anaesthesia, 45* (8), 669-71.
Borrelli, F., Capasso, R., Aviello, G., Pittler, M. H. & Izzo, A. A. (2005). "Effectiveness and safety of ginger in the treatment of pregnancy-induced nausea and vomiting." *Obstet Gynecol, 105* (4), 849-56. doi: 10.1097/01.aog.0000154890.47642.23.
Bryer, E. (2005). "A literature review of the effectiveness of ginger in alleviating mild-to-moderate nausea and vomiting of pregnancy." *J Midwifery Womens Health, 50* (1), e1-3. doi: 10.1016/j.jmwh.2004.08.023.
Carlson, Michelle J., Carolyn E Moore, Cynthia M Tsai, Robert J Shulman. & Bruno P Chumpitazi. (2014). "Child and parent perceived food-induced gastrointestinal symptoms and quality of life in children with functional gastrointestinal disorders." *Journal of the Academy of Nutrition and Dietetics, 114* (3), 403-413.
Chaiyakunapruk, N., Kitikannakorn, N., Nathisuwan, S., Leeprakobboon, K. & Leelasettagool, C. (2006). "The efficacy of ginger for the prevention of postoperative nausea and vomiting: a meta-analysis." *Am J Obstet Gynecol, 194* (1), 95-9. doi: 10.1016/j.ajog.2005.06.046.
Chiou, Eric. & Samuel Nurko. (2011). "Functional abdominal pain and irritable bowel syndrome in children and adolescents." *Therapy, 8* (3), 315.
Chrubasik, S., Pittler, M. H. & Roufogalis, B. D. (2005). "Zingiberis rhizoma: a comprehensive review on the ginger effect and efficacy profiles." *Phytomedicine, 12* (9), 684-701. doi: 10.1016/j.phymed.2004.07.009.
Chrubasik, Sigrun, Pittler, M. H. & Basil D. Roufogalis. (2005). *Zingiberis rhizoma: A comprehensive review on the ginger effect and efficacy profiles.*, Vol. *12.*
Cohen, M. (2007). "Traveller's 'funny tummy' - reviewing the evidence for complementary medicine." *Aust Fam Physician, 36* (5), 335-6.
Di Stefano, M., Miceli, E., Mazzocchi, S., Tana, P. & Corazza, G. R. (2005). "The role of gastric accommodation in the pathophysiology of functional dyspepsia." *Eur Rev Med Pharmacol Sci, 9*, (5 Suppl 1), 23-8.
Edwards, Trent, Craig Friesen. & Jennifer V Schurman. (2018). "Classification of pediatric functional gastrointestinal disorders related to abdominal pain using Rome III vs. Rome IV criterions." *BMC gastroenterology, 18* (1), 41.
Emma Westfall, Rachel. (2004). Use of anti-emetic herbs in pregnancy: Women's choices, and the question of safety and efficacy, *Complement Ther Nurs Midwifery, 10*(1):30-6. doi: 10.1016/S1353-6117(03)00057-X.
Ernst, E. & Pittler, M. H. (2000). "Efficacy of ginger for nausea and vomiting: a systematic review of randomized clinical trials." *Br J Anaesth, 84* (3), 367-71.
Fischer-Rasmussen, W., Kjaer, S. K., Dahl, C. & Asping, U. (1991). "Ginger treatment of hyperemesis gravidarum." *Eur J Obstet Gynecol Reprod Biol, 38* (1), 19-24.
Frisch, C., Hasenohrl, R. U., Mattern, C. M., Hacker, R. & Huston, J. P. (1995). "Blockade of lithium chloride-induced conditioned place aversion as a test for antiemetic agents: comparison of metoclopramide with combined extracts of Zingiber officinale and Ginkgo biloba." *Pharmacol Biochem Behav, 52* (2), 321-7.

Gaus, Kristen, Yue Huang, Dawn A. Israel, Susan L. Pendland, Bolanle A. Adeniyi. & Gail B. Mahady. (2009). "Standardized ginger (Zingiber officinale) extract reduces bacterial load and suppresses acute and chronic inflammation in Mongolian gerbils infected with cagAHelicobacter pylori." *Pharmaceutical biology, 47* (1), 92-98. doi: 10.1080/13880200802448690.

Ghayur, M. N. & Gilani, A. H. (2005). "Pharmacological basis for the medicinal use of ginger in gastrointestinal disorders." *Dig Dis Sci, 50* (10), 1889-97. doi: 10.1007/s10620-005-2957-2.

Ghayur, Muhammad Nabeel, Anwarul Hassan Gilani, Maria B Afridi. & Peter J Houghton. (2005). "Cardiovascular effects of ginger aqueous extract and its phenolic constituents are mediated through multiple pathways." *Vascular pharmacology, 43* (4), 234-241.

Gonlachanvit, S., Chen, Y. H., Hasler, W. L., Sun, W. M. & Owyang, C. (2003). "Ginger reduces hyperglycemia-evoked gastric dysrhythmias in healthy humans: possible role of endogenous prostaglandins." *J Pharmacol Exp Ther, 307* (3), 1098-103. doi: 10.1124/jpet.103.053421.

Govindarajan, V. S. (1982). "Ginger-chemistry, technology, and quality evaluation: part 2." *Crit Rev Food Sci Nutr, 17* (3), 189-258. doi: 10.1080/10408398209527348.

Grzanna, R., Lindmark, L. & Frondoza, C. G. (2005). "Ginger--an herbal medicinal product with broad anti-inflammatory actions." *J Med Food, 8* (2), 125-32. doi: 10.1089/jmf.2005.8.125.

Gupta, Y. K. & Sharma, M. (2001). "Reversal of pyrogallol-induced delay in gastric emptying in rats by ginger (Zingiber officinale)." *Methods Find Exp Clin Pharmacol, 23* (9), 501-3.

Haksar, A., Sharma, A., Chawla, R., Kumar, R., Arora, R., Singh, S., Prasad, J., Gupta, M., Tripathi, R. P., Arora, M. P., Islam, F. & Sharma, R. K. (2006). "Zingiber officinale exhibits behavioral radioprotection against radiation-induced CTA in a gender-specific manner." *Pharmacol Biochem Behav, 84* (2), 179-88. doi: 10.1016/j.pbb.2006.04.008.

Haniadka, R., Saldanha, E., Sunita, V., Palatty, P. L., Fayad, R. & Baliga, M. S. (2013). "A review of the gastroprotective effects of ginger (Zingiber officinale Roscoe)." *Food Funct, 4* (6), 845-55. doi: 10.1039/c3fo30337c.

Hickok, J. T., Roscoe, J. A., Morrow, G. R. & Ryan, J. L. (2007). "A Phase II/III Randomized, Placebo-Controlled, Double-Blind Clinical Trial of Ginger (Zingiber officinale) for Nausea Caused by Chemotherapy for Cancer: A Currently Accruing URCC CCOP Cancer Control Study." *Support Cancer Ther, 4* (4), 247-50. doi: 10.3816/SCT.2007.n.022.

Hollyer, T., Boon, H., Georgousis, A., Smith, M. & Einarson, A. (2002). "The use of CAM by women suffering from nausea and vomiting during pregnancy." *BMC Complement Altern Med, 2*, 5.

Hu, Ming-Luen, Christophan K Rayner, Keng-Liang Wu, Seng-Kee Chuah, Wei-Chen Tai, Yeh-Pin Chou, Yi-Chun Chiu, King-Wah Chiu. & Tsung-Hui Hu. (2011). "Effect of ginger on gastric motility and symptoms of functional dyspepsia." *World Journal of Gastroenterology: WJG, 17* (1), 105.

The International Agency for Research on Cancer (IARC). (1994). "Schistosomes, liver flukes and Helicobacter pylori." *IARC Working Group on the Evaluation of Carcinogenic Risks to Humans*. Lyon, 7-14 June 1994.

Jagetia, G., Baliga, M. & Venkatesh, P. (2004). "Ginger (Zingiber officinale Rosc.), a dietary supplement, protects mice against radiation-induced lethality: mechanism of action." *Cancer Biother Radiopharm, 19* (4), 422-35. doi: 10.1089/cbr.2004.19.422.

Janssen, P. L., Meyboom, S., van Staveren, W. A., de Vegt, F. & Katan, M. B. (1996). "Consumption of ginger (Zingiber officinale roscoe) does not affect ex vivo platelet thromboxane production in humans." *Eur J Clin Nutr, 50* (11), 772-4.

Johnson, Leonard R., James Christensen, Morton I Grossman, Eugene D Jacobson. & Stanley G Schultz. (1984). "Physiology of the gastrointestinal tract." *Journal of Pediatric Gastroenterology and Nutrition, 3* (1), 158.

Khushtar, M., Kumar, V., Javed, K. & Uma Bhandari. (2009). "Protective Effect of Ginger oil on Aspirin and Pylorus Ligation-Induced Gastric Ulcer model in Rats." *Indian journal of pharmaceutical sciences, 71* (5), 554-558. doi: 10.4103/0250-474X.58195.

Ko, J. K. & Leung, C. C. (2010). "Ginger extract and polaprezinc exert gastroprotective actions by anti-oxidant and growth factor modulating effects in rats." *J Gastroenterol Hepatol, 25* (12), 1861-8. doi: 10.1111/j.1440-1746.2010.06347.x.

Langner, E., Greifenberg, S. & Gruenwald, J. (1998). "Ginger: history and use." *Adv Ther, 15* (1), 25-44.

Lazzini, S., Polinelli, W., Riva, A., Morazzoni, P. & Bombardelli, E. (2016). "The effect of ginger (Zingiber officinalis) and artichoke (Cynara cardunculus) extract supplementation on gastric motility: a pilot randomized study in healthy volunteers." *Eur Rev Med Pharmacol Sci, 20* (1), 146-9.

Lee, Noel M. & Sumona Saha. (2011). "Nausea and vomiting of pregnancy." *Gastroenterology clinics of North America, 40* (2), 309-vii. doi: 10.1016/j.gtc.2011.03.009.

Lohsiriwat, Supatra, Mayurat Rukkiat, Reawika Chaikomin. & Somchai Leelakusolvong. (2010). *Effect of ginger on lower esophageal sphincter pressure.*, Vol. 93.

Lumb, A. B. (1993). "Mechanism of antiemetic effect of ginger." *Anaesthesia, 48* (12), 1118.

Lumb, A. B. (1994). "Effect of dried ginger on human platelet function." *Thromb Haemost, 71* (1), 110-1.

Mahady, G. B., Pendland, S. L., Yun, G. S., Lu, Z. Z. & Stoia, A. (2003). "Ginger (Zingiber officinale Roscoe) and the gingerols inhibit the growth of Cag A+ strains of Helicobacter pylori." *Anticancer Res, 23* (5a), 3699-702.

Manusirivithaya, S., Sripramote, M., Tangjitgamol, S., Sheanakul, C., Leelahakorn, S., Thavaramara, T. & Tangcharoenpanich, K. (2004). "Antiemetic effect of ginger in gynecologic oncology patients receiving cisplatin." *Int J Gynecol Cancer, 14* (6), 1063-9. doi: 10.1111/j.1048-891X.2004.14603.x.

Meltzer, Donna I. (2000). "Complementary therapies for nausea and vomiting in early pregnancy." *Family Practice, 17* (6), 570-573. doi: 10.1093/fampra/17.6.570.

Micklefield, G. H., Redeker, Y., Meister, V., Jung, O., Greving, I. & May, B. (1999). "Effects of ginger on gastroduodenal motility." *Int J Clin Pharmacol Ther, 37* (7), 341-6.

Moneret-Vautrin, D. A., Morisset, M., Lemerdy, P., Croizier, A. & Kanny, G. (2002). "Food allergy and IgE sensitization caused by spices: CICBAA data (based on 589 cases of food allergy)." *Allerg Immunol (Paris), 34* (4), 135-40.

Nakazawa, Takahiro. & Keisuke Ohsawa. (2002). "Metabolism of [6]-gingerol in rats." *Life sciences, 70* (18), 2165-2175.

Parveen, Abida, Bushra Parveen, Rabea Parveen. & Sayeed Ahmad. (2015). "Challenges and guidelines for clinical trial of herbal drugs." *Journal of pharmacy & bioallied sciences, 7* (4), 329-333. doi: 10.4103/0975-7406.168035.

Pfeiffer, E., Heuschmid, F. F., Kranz, S. & Metzler, M. (2006). "Microsomal hydroxylation and glucuronidation of [6]-gingerol." *J Agric Food Chem, 54* (23), 8769-74. doi: 10.1021/jf062235l.

Pike, Andrea, Holly Etchegary, Marshall Godwin, Farah McCrate, John Crellin, Maria Mathews, Rebecca Law, Leigh Anne Newhook. & Jody Kinden. (2013). "Use of natural health products in children: qualitative analysis of parents' experiences." *Canadian Family Physician, 59* (8), e372-e378.

Portnoi, G., Chng, L. A., Karimi-Tabesh, L., Koren, G., Tan, M. P. & Einarson, A. (2003). "Prospective comparative study of the safety and effectiveness of ginger for the treatment of nausea and vomiting in pregnancy." *Am J Obstet Gynecol, 189* (5), 1374-7.

Prakash, U. N. & Srinivasan, K. (2010). "Gastrointestinal protective effect of dietary spices during ethanol-induced oxidant stress in experimental rats." *Appl Physiol Nutr Metab, 35* (2), 134-41. doi: 10.1139/h09-133.

Qian, Q. H., Yue, W., Chen, W. H., Yang, Z. H., Liu, Z. T. & Wang, Y. X. (2010). "Effect of gingerol on substance P and NK1 receptor expression in a vomiting model of mink." *Chin Med J (Engl), 123* (4), 478-84.

Quinla, J. D. & Hill, D. A. (2003). "Nausea and vomiting of pregnancy." *Am Fam Physician, 68* (1), 121-8.

Reddy, A. C. & Lokesh, B. R. (1992). "Studies on spice principles as antioxidants in the inhibition of lipid peroxidation of rat liver microsomes." *Mol Cell Biochem, 111* (1-2), 117-24.

Rong, X., Peng, G., Suzuki, T., Yang, Q., Yamahara, J. & Li, Y. (2009). "A 35-day gavage safety assessment of ginger in rats." *Regul Toxicol Pharmacol, 54* (2), 118-23. doi: 10.1016/j.yrtph.2009.03.002.

Seynaeve, C., De Mulder, P. H. & Verweij, J. (1991). "Pathophysiology of cytotoxic drug-induced emesis: far from crystal-clear." *Pharm Weekbl Sci, 13* (1), 1-6.

Shanmugam, K. R., Ramakrishna, C. H., Mallikarjuna, K. & Reddy, K. S. (2010). "Protective effect of ginger against alcohol-induced renal damage and antioxidant enzymes in male albino rats." *Indian J Exp Biol, 48* (2), 143-9.

Sharma, A., Haksar, A., Chawla, R., Kumar, R., Arora, R., Singh, S., Prasad, J., Islam, F., Arora, M. P. & Kumar Sharma, R. (2005). "Zingiber officinale Rosc. modulates gamma radiation-induced conditioned taste aversion." *Pharmacol Biochem Behav, 81* (4), 864-70. doi: 10.1016/j.pbb.2005.06.012.

Sharma, S. S. & Gupta, Y. K. (1998). "Reversal of cisplatin-induced delay in gastric emptying in rats by ginger (Zingiber officinale)." *J Ethnopharmacol, 62* (1), 49-55.

Sharma, S. S., Kochupillai, V., Gupta, S. K., Seth, S. D. & Gupta, Y. K. (1997). "Antiemetic efficacy of ginger (Zingiber officinale) against cisplatin-induced emesis in dogs." *J Ethnopharmacol, 57* (2), 93-6.

Shukla, Yogeshwer. & Madhulika Singh. (2007). "Cancer preventive properties of ginger: a brief review." *Food and chemical toxicology, 45* (5), 683-690.

Siddaraju, M. N. & Dharmesh, S. M. (2007). "Inhibition of gastric H+, K+-ATPase and Helicobacter pylori growth by phenolic antioxidants of Zingiber officinale." *Mol Nutr Food Res, 51* (3), 324-32. doi: 10.1002/mnfr.200600202.

Singletary, Keith. (2010). "Ginger: An Overview of Health Benefits." *Nutrition Today, 45*, 171-183. doi: 10.1097/NT.0b013e3181ed3543.

Smith, C., Crowther, C., Willson, K., Hotham, N. & McMillian, V. (2004). "A randomized controlled trial of ginger to treat nausea and vomiting in pregnancy." *Obstet Gynecol, 103* (4), 639-45. doi: 10.1097/01.AOG.0000118307.19798.ec.

Srivas, K. C. (1984). "Effects of aqueous extracts of onion, garlic and ginger on platelet aggregation and metabolism of arachidonic acid in the blood vascular system: *in vitro* study." *Prostaglandins Leukot Med, 13* (2), 227-35.

Srivastava, K. C. (1986). "Isolation and effects of some ginger components of platelet aggregation and eicosanoid biosynthesis." *Prostaglandins Leukot Med, 25* (2-3), 187-98.

Suekawa, M., Ishige, A., Yuasa, K., Sudo, K., Aburada, M. & Hosoya, E. (1984). "Pharmacological studies on ginger. I. Pharmacological actions of pungent constitutents, (6)-gingerol and (6)-shogaol." *J Pharmacobiodyn, 7* (11), 836-48.

Surh, Young-Joon. & Sang Sup Lee. (1994). "Enzymic reduction of [6]-gingerol, a major pungent principle of ginger, in the cell-free preparation of rat liver." *Life Sciences, 54* (19), PL321-PL326. doi: https://doi.org/10.1016/0024-3205(94)00602-4.

Tavlan, A., Tuncer, S., Erol, A., Reisli, R., Aysolmaz, G. & Otelcioglu, S. (2006). "Prevention of postoperative nausea and vomiting after thyroidectomy: combined antiemetic treatment with dexamethasone and ginger versus dexamethasone alone." *Clin Drug Investig, 26* (4), 209-14. doi: 10.2165/00044011-200626040-00005.

Thompson, H. J. & Potter, P. J. (2006). "Review: ginger prevents 24 hour postoperative nausea and vomiting." *Evid Based Nurs, 9* (3), 80.

van Tilburg, M. A., Palsson, O. S., Levy, R. L., Feld, A. D., Turner, M. J., Drossman, D. A. & Whitehead, W. E. (2008). "Complementary and alternative medicine use and cost in functional bowel disorders: a six month prospective study in a large HMO." *BMC Complement Altern Med, 8*, 46. doi: 10.1186/1472-6882-8-46.

van Tilburg, M. A., Palsson, O. S., Ringel, Y. & Whitehead, W. E. (2014). "Is ginger effective for the treatment of irritable bowel syndrome? A double blind randomized controlled pilot trial." *Complement Ther Med, 22* (1), 17-20. doi: 10.1016/j.ctim.2013.12.015.

Varni, James W., Cristiane B Bendo, Jolanda Denham, Robert J Shulman, Mariella M Self, Deborah A Neigut, Samuel Nurko, Ashish S Patel, James P Franciosi. & Miguel Saps. (2015). "PedsQL™ Gastrointestinal Symptoms Scales and Gastrointestinal Worry Scales in pediatric patients with functional and organic gastrointestinal diseases in comparison to healthy controls." *Quality of Life Research, 24* (2), 363-378.

Vutyavanich, T., Kraisarin, T. & Ruangsri, R. (2001). "Ginger for nausea and vomiting in pregnancy: randomized, double-masked, placebo-controlled trial." *Obstet Gynecol, 97* (4), 577-82.

Weidner, M. S. & Sigwart, K. (2000). "The safety of a ginger extract in the rat." *J Ethnopharmacol, 73* (3), 513-20.

Wilkinson, J. M. (2000). "Effect of ginger tea on the fetal development of Sprague-Dawley rats." *Reprod Toxicol, 14* (6), 507-12.

Yamahara, J., Mochizuki, M., Rong, H. Q., Matsuda, H. & Fujimura, H. (1988). "The anti-ulcer effect in rats of ginger constituents." *J Ethnopharmacol, 23* (2-3), 299-304.

Yoshikawa, T., Naito, Y., Kishi, A., Tomii, T., Kaneko, T., Iinuma, S., Ichikawa, H., Yasuda, M., Takahashi, S. & Kondo, M. (1993). "Role of active oxygen, lipid peroxidation, and antioxidants in the pathogenesis of gastric mucosal injury induced by indomethacin in rats." *Gut, 34* (6), 732-737.

Yuki, Mika, Yoshinori Komazawa, Yoshiya Kobayashi, Maho Kusunoki, Yoshiko Takahashi, Sayaka Nakashima, Goichi Uno, Isao Ikuma, Toshihiro Shizuku. & Yoshikazu Kinoshita. (2015). "Effects of Daikenchuto on abdominal bloating accompanied by chronic constipation: A prospective, single-center randomized open trial." *Current Therapeutic Research, 77*, 58-62.

Zick, S. M., Djuric, Z., Ruffin, M. T., Litzinger, A. J., Normolle, D. P., Alrawi, S., Feng, M. R. & Brenner, D. E. (2008). "Pharmacokinetics of 6-gingerol, 8-gingerol, 10-gingerol, and 6-shogaol and conjugate metabolites in healthy human subjects." *Cancer Epidemiol Biomarkers Prev, 17* (8), 1930-6. doi: 10.1158/1055-9965.epi-07-2934.

Zick, S. M., Ruffin, M. T., Lee, J., Normolle, D. P., Siden, R., Alrawi, S. & Brenner, D. E. (2009). "Phase II trial of encapsulated ginger as a treatment for chemotherapy-induced nausea and vomiting." *Support Care Cancer, 17* (5), 563-72. doi: 10.1007/s00520-008-0528-8.

Chapter 2

Potential Benefits of Ginger in Maintenance of Oral Health

C. Pushpalatha*, Kavita Kamondur and Arshiya Shakir

Department of Pediatric and Preventive Dentistry, Faculty of Dental Science, Ramaiah University of Applied Sciences, Bengaluru, India

Abstract

Ginger rhizomes or Zingiberofficinale is a perennial crop grown in tropical and subtropical regions worldwide. It has been used as traditional medicine for 2500 years to alleviate headaches, cold and gastrointestinal disorders. It is also used as an alternative medicine to treat rheumatological, musculoskeletal, and dyslipidemia conditions [1]. Minerals, vitamins, and phytochemicals are abundant in ginger. Recently, ginger has received a lot of interest in dentistry to avoid tooth problems. Ginger has no toxicity hence it is regarded as safe (GRAS) by the US Food and Drug Administration [2]. The polyphenolic ketones or Gingerols present in ginger are mainly responsible for pharmacological effects such as antioxidant, anti-inflammatory, and antimicrobial activities. It was first reported in the early 1980s that ginger has anti-inflammatory activity since it has the potential to inhibit prostaglandins synthesis. Gingerols and Shogaols present in ginger exhibit pharmacological characteristics that are similar to dual-acting non-steroidal anti-inflammatory medications. The ginger antioxidant activity is responsible for protection against radiation toxicity and lethality. Ginger exhibits antibacterial activity against Streptococcus mutans and Streptococcus sanguinis. Since ginger has a wide range of

---

*Corresponding Author's Email: drpushpalatha29@gmail.com.

In: Ginger and its Health Benefits
Editor: Isla Kermode
ISBN: 978-1-68507-695-5
© 2022 Nova Science Publishers, Inc.

pharmacotherapeutic characteristics, it has been used to treat oral diseases [3-5]. This chapter highlights the composition and properties of ginger, oral application, and the future scope of ginger in dentistry.

Keywords: Ginger, Oral Application, Antibacterial Activity, Anti-inflammatory

1. Introduction

Medicinal plant-based treatment is as ancient as mankind. The primitive plants with established medicinal values are mainly used due to their definitive physiological actions on the individuals. These physiological actions are mainly because of bioactive constituents present in the plants namely phenolic substances, flavonoids, alkaloids, and tannins. Medicinal plants have been used for ages as chemotherapeutic agents mostly for the presence of these bioactive components [6]. Ginger has been shown to help in food digestion, flu, colds, and nausea prevention. Ginger is used in a variety of forms, including ginger slices, grated ginger, ginger paste, ginger juice, and ginger oil. The increasing issue of resistance towards synthetic antimicrobials has rekindled curiosity in natural products as an alternative therapy. The research focusing on the identification of newer antimicrobial drugs for inhibition of microbial biofilm led to the discovery of different natural products that are effective against oral diseases like dental caries, gingival and periodontal diseases [1]. The natural drug molecules are considered effective antibacterial agents against different types of oral pathogens. Reports are showing that essential oils act as an effective antibacterial agent. Even naturally derived aromatic molecules are widely used for oral care as an alternative therapy. Among the medicinal plants, ginger has been used for various medicinal purposes since the ancient period. It is composed of nearly 1200 species with 53 genera. In 1807 ginger was officially coined as Zingiberofficinale by William Roscoe, an English botanist [7]. Where Zingiber refers to "shaped like a deer's antlers" and officinale means rhizomes medicinal qualities. Ginger is a tropical and subtropical crop cultivated all over the world. It is sold in the international market in various forms like fresh or dried products, as an extract, as powder form, tablets, and tea bags. India is the major ginger producer followed by China, Nepal, and Thailand. Ginger has a therapeutic role in the prevention of dental diseases by modifying biological activities.

The ginger constituents mainly Gingerols and Shogaols are essential for the therapeutic effects. Ginger can be used individually or combined with other natural products to bring the desired therapeutic effects. This assertion has been supported by recent scientific studies. In terms of oral health, ginger has been shown to have an inhibitory effect on the development of microorganisms that cause tooth decay. It acts as a dental anesthetic drug and can also aid in dentine remineralization. Ginger's antiplaque and oral deodorizing properties have also been widely researched. Ginger toothpaste and tooth powder assist to keep teeth clean and free of tartar and caries [12]. Ginger is added into different formulations to obtain the ginger benefit in the prevention of oral diseases. This chapter summarizes the properties of ginger and its oral application.

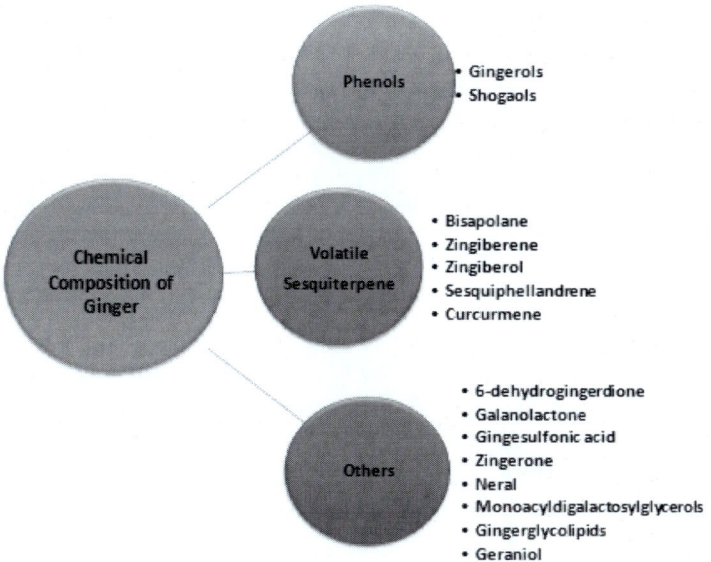

Figure 1. Chemical Composition of Ginger.

2. Chemical Composition of Ginger

Ginger is a rich source of active ingredients such as phenolic compounds (Gingerol and Shogoal), Volatile oils (Zingiberene, Zingiberol), sesquiterpene hydrocarbons, oleoresins, and Diarylheptanoids (Gingerenones A and B)

(Figure 1). Sesquiterpene hydrocarbons are the most often discovered terpene components. The combination of terpenes and oleoresin active ingredients is called ginger oil. Ginger constitutes volatile oils approximately 1% to 3% and non-volatile pungent components called oleoresin. Ginger also has a high content of minerals, vitamins, carbohydrates, protein, fats, soluble and insoluble fibers, and phytochemicals. Gingerols exhibit pharmacological activities such as antioxidant, anti-inflammatory, and antimicrobial activities.

3. Properties of Ginger

Alkylated gingerols extracted from ethanol and n-hexane extracts of ginger were shown to possess antibacterial, anti-tumorigenic, antioxidant, and anti-inflammatory actions (Figure 2). It also has antibacterial activity against Staphylococcus aureus and Streptococcus pyogenes that is higher than that of commercially available antibiotics.

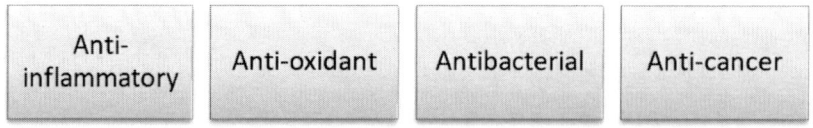

Figure 2. Properties of Ginger.

3.1. Anti-inflammatory Property

Ginger has been found to have inhibitory effects on prostaglandins synthesis. The anti-inflammatory activity was reported for the first time in the early 1980s [8]. Ginger's Gingerdiones and Shogaols have pharmacological effects that are similar to non-steroidal anti-inflammatory medications (NSAIDs). Because ginger has fewer negative effects than traditional NSAIDs, it is now being researched as a new family of anti-inflammatory solutions [9].

The mechanism by which Ginger acts is found to be by prevention of arachidonic acid breakdown via the cyclooxygenase and lipoxygenase pathways [10]. The stimulation of many genes implicated in the inflammatory response, as well as genes encrypting cytokines, chemokines, and the inducible COX-2 (enzyme cyclooxygenase-2), was found to be inhibited by ginger.

The volatile oils in ginger can impact both cell-mediated immune responses and nonspecific T lymphocyte proliferation. Allowing them to modify lymphocyte and cellular immune responses. As a result, many have positive benefits in a variety of clinical situations, including chronic inflammation and autoimmune disorders [11].

3.2. Antioxidant Property

Ginger has a rich source of antioxidants mainly ginger essential oil and oleoresins which exhibit 1, 1 Diphenyl, 2 picrylhydrazyl (DPPH) free radical activity of scavenging in a concentration-dependent manner. The Ginger extract's antioxidant activity is responsible for its protection against radiation toxicity and lethality [12], against a variety of toxic chemicals such as carbon tetrachloride and cisplatin [13, 14], and as an anti-ulcer drug [15]. With relation to Fe^{3+}, ginger has a strong chelate-forming ability, stopping hydroxyl radicals from forming, which are recognized as lipid peroxidation inducers [16, 17]. Polyphenols, tannins, and flavonoids are considered the main antioxidant components of ginger.

3.3. Antibacterial Property

According to research using gas chromatography-mass spectrometry, ginger essential oil and oleoresins include significant levels of phenolic chemicals, which are responsible for antibacterial activity (Figure 3). The antibacterial activity of ginger extract has various mechanisms. The antibacterial activity against oral pathogens mainly Streptococcus mutans is as follows. Ginger extract affects the sucrose dependent (SD) and sucrose independent (SI) adherence of Streptococcus mutans. Ginger extract blocks the enzyme glucosyltransferases (GTPase), which converts sucrose into sticky glucans, allowing Streptococcus mutans to adhere to the tooth surface. In the presence of ginger extract, the index of hydrophobicity was also significantly reduced. Due to reduced hydrophobic interactions between the cells and the surface, bacteria were unable to adhere to the surface. Biofilm formation was prevented as a result of these factors. The function of a variety of enzymes engaged in physiological activities such as glycolysis, cell perseverance, and intracellular and extracellular polysaccharide synthesis was impaired by ginger extract, potentially killing the Streptococcus mutans. The ginger extract also showed suppression of protein expression. In the presence of Ginger extract, the whole set of pathogenic genes relA, brpA, gtfC, and comDE were downregulated. Gene relA is involved in Streptococcus mutans oxidative stress and acid tolerance pathways, whereas gene brpA is important for biofilm production and structural integrity. As a result, downregulating these genes reduces virulence expression. The regulatory gene comDE is part of the Streptococcus mutans quorum-sensing cascade, and its downregulation weakens the organism's internal communication system [18]. Gingerol and shogaol from the rhizome of the ginger plant have antibacterial properties against anaerobic bacteria that cause periodontal disease in the oral cavity [19].

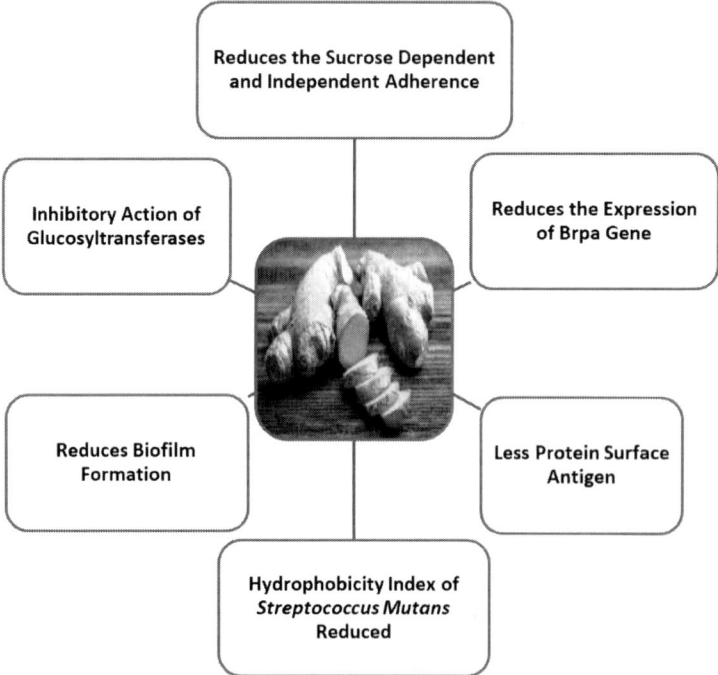

Figure 3. Antibacterial Action of Ginger.

3.4. Anti-Cancer Property and Radioprotective Action

The anticancer properties of ginger components have been widely researched [12]. By triggering apoptosis, upregulating tumor suppressor genes, and inhibiting angiogenic factors (vascular endothelial growth factor), ginger can help to limit tumor development and proliferation. Components such as 6-gingerol, 6-shogaol, 6-paradol, zingerone, and zerumbone have been found to have significant anticancer effects through various studies [20, 21]. In a dose-dependent way, ginger essential oil suppressed mutagenicity produced by direct-acting mutagens. By inhibiting the transcription factor NF-kb, ginger root extract and its major polyphenolic component demonstrate anti-mutagenic action in a variety of cell types. In-vitro studies comparing the ginger extract and 6-gingerol show that 6-gingerol has stronger anti-mutagenic activity than ginger extract mainly through regulating the proliferation of YYT cancer cells, Microsatellite instability endothelial cells, and angiogenesis suppression [22]. Even though ginger has anti-cancer property it can even be used in patients with radiotherapy due to its radio-protective action. The phytochemical action of ginger substitutes like dehydrogingerone and zingerone protects normal tissues from tumoricidal effects and prevents gamma radiation-induced illness [20]. This property is also confirmed in a study done by Rashmi et al., where ginger extracts if given before radiotherapy reduced glutathione reductase, glutathione peroxidase enzyme activities, and also lipid peroxidation thus leading to radio-protective action [21].

4. Formulations of Ginger

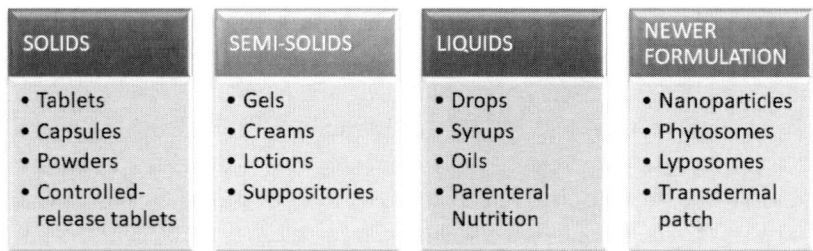

Figure 4. Formulations of Ginger.

Different types of medication formulations can be administered to a patient in various forms, including solids such as tablets, capsules, powders, and controlled-release tablets; semisolids such as gels, creams, lotions, and suppositories; and liquids such as drops, syrups, oils, and parenteral nutrition (Figure 4). Formulation administration depends on certain criteria, like patient's condition, age, gender, drug release rate, and health state, all of which are unique to distinct routes of administration. With newer advances in the pharmacodynamics of drug administration, ginger formulations are also available like nanoparticles, phytosomes, liposomes, and transdermal patches [23].

5. Systemic Applications of Ginger

Ginger is used in the treatment of ulcers as it increases mucin secretion. Ginger antagonizes the 5-HT3 receptor and has an antiserotonergic action because of components like gingerols, shogaols, and galanolactone, as well as diterpenoid. This might be crucial for preventing nausea and vomiting after surgery [20, 21]. Ginger's antioxidant properties combat aging in people [12]. Gingerol extract has shown to be a promising source for the formulation of novel medications mainly as a chemotherapeutic agent for the management of oral diseases. Some studies have shown that giving ginger to rats for a month protects them from ethanol-induced hepatotoxicity. It has also been discovered to have important adjuvant benefits in patients with acute and chronic renal failure, preventing disease development and delaying the need for renal replacement treatment [24]. Ginger can be used in motion sickness, morning sickness, unsettled stomach, diarrhea, nausea, and lack of appetite caused during cancer therapy or surgery [25]. Ginger has anti-colon cancer properties. Ginger enhances the effects of warfarin. Ginger should not be used in patients who receive an oral anticoagulant since it may raise the danger of bleeding or intensify the result of the medication [25]. Ginger has a significant antihyperglycemic effect. Ginger lowers fasting blood sugar and hemoglobin A1c in Type 2 diabetes, as well as boosting GLUT4 expression, which increases insulin-dependent glucose absorption. Ginger's hypoglycemic impact is due to its ability to suppress oxidative stress and anti-inflammatory effects [21]. Ginger has bronchodilator properties, making it useful in the management of upper respiratory tract infections, cough, and bronchitis [25]. Ginger syrup is used as a therapy for the bronchial effects of respiratory issues, cough, and as an adjuvant in the management of SARS-CoV-2 [23].

6. Oral Applications of Ginger

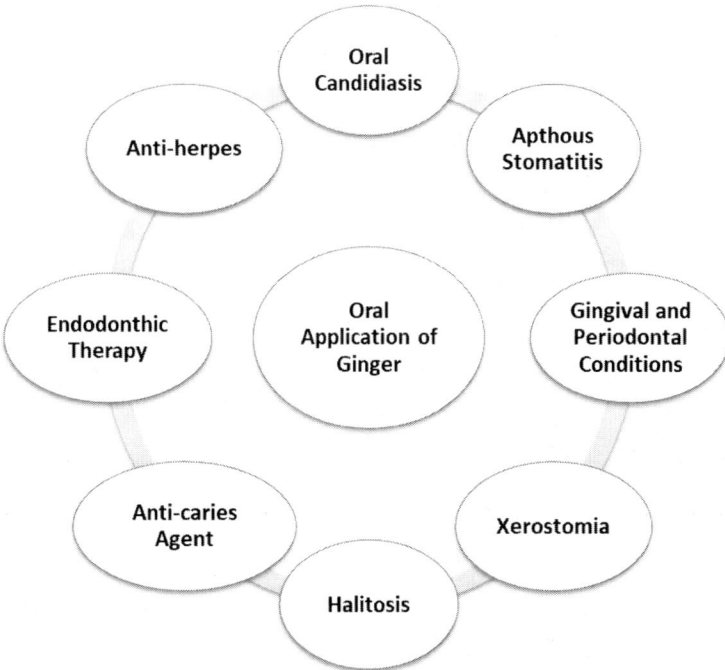

Figure 5. Oral Applications of Ginger.

6.1. Oral Candidiasis

Oral candidiasis is a common fungal infection seen orally. It is a disorder where Candida albicans deposits on the mucosal lining of the oral cavity causing white lesions on the mucosal surface. The synthetic topical and systemic antifungal therapies cause drug resistance which reduces their clinical effectiveness. Hence ginger was studied for antifungal activity against Candida albicans which is a causative agent for oral candidiasis. A study done by Khalaf et al. showed that the alcoholic extracts of ginger were effective against Candida albicans suggesting it can be used in the treatment of oral candidiasis. This study proved that the ginger roots contain a substance called CMUAC 130 which acts as an inhibitory effect on the biofilm formation of Candida albicans [9]. This antifungal activity for the treatment of oral candidiasis was further confirmed by comparing ginger and other antifungal medicines like fluconazole, amphotericin B, and nystatin for the prevention of Candida albicans colonization. Results showed concentrations of 50, 10, and 10 mg/mL of the crude extract have inhibition zone up to 18, 21, and 25 mm [4, 5]. Hence ginger can act as a topical antifungal agent when incorporated into oral medications.

6.2. Apthous Stomatitis

Aphthous Stomatitis is a frequent pathological disease affecting the oral cavity. It is a benign disorder characterized by oral ulcers that appear all over the mouth. The ulcers are tiny, circular, and numerous [12]. Ginger has antipyretic property hence can be used as an analgesic. In a study, it was proved that when dried ginger rhizome (DGR) was applied on aphthous ulcers it gave an analgesic effect. DGR has been proven to be a strong agonist of TRPV1 channels (Transient receptor potential cation channel subfamily V member 1) which provide a warm sensation by sensitizing sensory endings in inflamed ulcer tissues before sensitizing to pain, which is believed to be the cause of ulcer pain alleviation. The same study concludes that DGR can be used in aphthous stomatitis treatment as analgesia, promoting wound healing and for immune suppression [13]. This theory was proven in a study by Parya et al., in which a ginger-containing mucoadhesive system was examined for its efficiency in the treatment of aphthous stomatitis, the results revealed a marked reduction in discomfort and a major drop in the inflammatory zone [14].

6.3. Gingival and Periodontal Conditions

Gingivitis occurs when subgingival bacteria interfere with gingival tissue and induce inflammation of the barrier function of the sulcular epithelium. The pathologic alterations in gingivitis are connected to the oral sulcus and the tooth attaching bacterial pathogens [15]. These pathogens are Prevotella intermedia, Porphyromonas gingivalis, and Porphyromonas endodontalis which are responsible for gingivitis and periodontitis [16] since ginger is known to have antimicrobial properties. Hence it can be used in mouthwashes and in powder form to treat gingival and periodontal conditions. They work by suppressing COX-1 and COX-2 enzymes, which reduce prostaglandin biosynthesis and decrease the proliferation of anaerobic Gram-negative periodontal bacteria such as Prevotella intermedia, Porphyromonas endodontalis, and Porphyromonas gingivalis [15] these findings are confirmed in a randomized control study done by Anshula et al., which showed a significant reduction in both plaque score and gingival index in children after using ginger mouthwashes [16]. Similar findings were observed in which ginger mouthwashes were effective in patients with gingivitis when compared with chlorhexidine mouthwashes [15]. A study by Pallavi et al. compared the effects of ginger and ibuprofen on pain and gingival inflammation after open flap debridement. During open flap debridement, the dried ginger powder was shown equally effective to Ibuprofen in decreasing pain and gingival inflammation [17]. A review of the literature reveals that ginger extracts have antibacterial action against the most common periodontal infections. Hence, they can be used to prevent and cure periodontal illnesses instead of chemical antiseptics [18].

6.4. Xerostomia

Xerostomia means dry mouth, a condition with a decrease in salivation which leads to dry mouth [19]. Studies confirm that ginger has prokinetic activity and cholinergic effects. The mechanism by which ginger increases salivary secretion is through parasympathetic activity on the postsynaptic M3 receptors and suppressive effect on presynaptic muscarinic autoreceptors [8]. Hence based on this mechanism of action ginger sprays were used in diabetic xerostomic patients where ginger sprays rapidly increased the patients' saliva and satisfaction [19]. When ginger capsules were administered to patients with xerostomia after radiotherapy of the head and neck region, similar results were observed. Ginger also relieved xerostomia signs by enhancing the rate of salivary production in the patients [26, 27].

6.5. During Endodontic Therapy

The goal of tooth endodontic therapy is to remove causative microorganisms from the root canal, dentinal tubules, and periapical region of the tooth. Enterococcus faecalis is a resistant microorganism and plays a significant role in root canal treatment failure. Chemical cleaning of the canals using endodontic irrigation solutions is one of the most essential procedures in root canal therapy. As ginger has antibacterial activity, it was used for irrigating the canals, the result showed that ginger extract has potential antimicrobial action against root canal pathogens [28]. Similar findings were also seen when ginger was utilized as an intracanal medicament to decrease Candida albicans, Enterococcus faecalis, Escherichia coli, and their endotoxins in the root canals. The findings revealed that ginger-based intracanal medicament was effective in removing germs from the root canal and lowering endotoxins [29]. Fathima malik evaluated the inhibitory effect of ginger extract on bacteria isolated from endodontic canals, the bacteria isolated were Lactobacillus species, Viridans Streptococcus, Staphylococcus species, and Prevotella intermedia. The study also revealed that ginger oil is most effective when compared with green tea and amoxicillin in the prevention of endodontic infections [30].

6.6. As Anti-Caries Agent

Ginger has many advantages when used as an individual agent in the form of toothpaste where it has an anti-caries activity, increases the hardness of dentine, remineralization potential, reduces sensitivity, and can be used as a polishing agent after oral prophylaxis [12]. Dental caries is one of the most progressing diseases of the oral cavity [31]. Streptococcus sanguinis and Streptococcus mutans are two organisms that are mostly associated with dental caries [12]. The antibacterial activities of ginger extracts against these bacteria were examined, and the findings indicated that methanol and ethyl acetate extracts of ginger possess antimicrobial activity against Streptococcus mutans and Streptococcus sanguinis. Ginger's anti-biofilm, anti-adhesion, and bactericidal activities reduce the incidence of dental caries [31]. A similar finding was observed in a study by Jain et al. [32] where the antibacterial activity of an organic solvent-based ginger extract against Streptococcus mutans was the highest. Ginger was also assessed to check for remineralizing ability and a study by Celic et al. showed ginger has promising results of tooth remineralization [33]. Another study suggested that zerumbone et al., one of the active components of ginger, had a minimum inhibitory concentration of 250 g/mL and a minimum bactericidal concentration of 500 g/mL against Streptococcus mutans, indicating that it may be utilized as a preventative anti-cariogenic agent [34]. Ginger's ability to modulate dentin stiffness and hardness was also investigated. The treatment effects using ginger (oil), sodium hypochlorite, and Ethylenediaminetetraacetic acid were tested, and the results showed that ginger (oil) reduced dentin micro-hardness compared to others [35]. Several studies have been conducted to check if herbal products can replace the chemical product to attain remineralization potential. Ginger, rosemary, and sodium fluoride were compared on incipient white spot lesions and the results confirmed that ginger could inhibit demineralization and promote remineralization of white spot lesions in the enamel and can serve as a treatment option for the management of white spot lesions. Ginger showed remineralization potential at 0.5% concentration. The free calcium ions needed for remineralization were provided from within ginger itself [36]. A similar study by Azhar et al., showed that herbal products like tea tree oil, ginger, and grape seed had remineralization properties [37].

6.7. Anti-Herpes Activity

Researchers have reported the anti-viral action of ginger and can be used to treat herpes infection of the oral cavity [38]. HSV-1, also known as Herpes simplex virus type 1, is a common infection in both children and adults usually associated with primary infections that manifest clinically as herpes labialis or primary herpetic gingivostomatitis [39]. The ginger essential oil has an antiviral effect where it prevents virus adsorption before it enters the host cell. The essential oil disrupts the virion envelop structure. Pretreatment with essential oil causes viral to envelop disruption. The essential oil's lipophilic component interacts with the lipid membrane disrupting the integrity of the virus [12]. HSV showed sensitivity to several essential oils and their components where the ginger constituents interact with HSV particles thus limiting cell adsorption. Ginger oils possess direct virucidal action and prevent intracellular multiplication. Essential oils are most vulnerable to acyclovir-resistant HSV strains since their mechanism is entirely different from that of synthetic drugs [40].

6.8. Halitosis Management

Halitosis/Bad breath is a foul or disagreeable odor originating from the oral region during exhaling breath. Since ginger has antimicrobial properties, it is used in mouthwashes to reduce halitosis [12]. It is shown that when a mixture of herbal products containing ginger is used as mouthwashes in such patients, there was a reduction in halitosis. This action is achieved due to the presence of phytochemicals in the [41].

7. Toxicity of Ginger

Ginger was discovered to have the most antibacterial activity of all-natural dietary sources. It is a non-toxic natural substance and classified as "generally regarded as safe" by US Food and Drug Administration. The oil component of ginger consists of a series of polyphenol ketones with various pharmacological activities [42]. Humans can consume up to 2mg of ginger in moderate doses. After oral intake, the phytoconstituents of ginger, gingerol, and shogaol, are effectively absorbed and bio-transformed [12]. Ginger extract formulation containing 8% total gingerols fed to rats to the maximum dose of 2000 mg/kg showed no acute toxicity. There were no toxic effects to a maximum dose of 1000 mg/kg on repeated administration for 28 days to the rats. In a study after administration of ginger extract for 10days to pregnant rats at different concentrations of 100, 333, and 1000 mg/kg at the organogenesis period showed no maternal or developmental toxicity [43].

Conclusion

In conclusion, ginger has a wide range of pharmacological actions. The exact mechanism of each action, however, remains unclear. Despite a lack of mechanistic data, ginger appears to be safe and is nevertheless frequently used for dental and other therapeutic purposes. The herbal formulations with active ingredients and their molecular interactions are poorly understood, which makes product standardization difficult. Although large-scale clinical trials are needed to confirm its use in medicine and dentistry safely, there is currently inadequate data to prove its efficacy and dosages in the treatment of oral diseases.

References

[1] Lippolis V, Irurhe O, Porricelli AC, Cortese M, Schena R, Imafidon T, Oluwadun A, Pascale M. Natural co-occurrence of aflatoxins and ochratoxin A in ginger (Zingiberofficinale) from Nigeria. *Food Control.* 2017 Mar 1;73:1061-7.

[2] Ali BH, Blunden G, Tanira MO, Nemmar A. Some phytochemical, pharmacological and toxicological properties of ginger (Zingiberofficinale Roscoe): a review of recent research. *Food and Chemical Toxicology.* 2008 Feb 1;46(2):409-20.

[3] Semwal RB, Semwal DK, Combrinck S, Viljoen AM. Gingerols and shogaols: Important nutraceutical principles from ginger. *Phytochemistry.* 2015 Sep 1;117:554-68.

[4] Singh G, Kapoor IP, Singh P, de Heluani CS, de Lampasona MP, Catalan CA. Chemistry, antioxidant and antimicrobial investigations on essential oil and oleoresins of Zingiberofficinale. *Food and Chemical Toxicology.* 2008 Oct 1;46(10):3295-302.

[5] PR SA, Prakash J. Chemical composition and antioxidant properties of ginger root (Zingiberofficinale). *Journal of Medicinal Plants Research.* 2010 Dec 18;4(24):2674-9.

[6] Komandur K, Pushpalatha C, Deveswaran R. Formulation of a ginger extract liquid bandage and in-vitro assessment of physical and chemical characteristics. In *AIP Conference Proceedings 2020 Oct 5* (Vol. 2274, No. 1, p. 050009). AIP Publishing LLC.

[7] Amin A, Hamza AA. Effects of Roselle and Ginger on cisplatin-induced reproductive toxicity in rats. *Asian Journal of Andrology.* 2006 Sep;8(5):607-12.

[8] Park M, Bae J, Lee DS. Antibacterial activity of [10]-gingerol and [12]-gingerol isolated from ginger rhizome against periodontal bacteria. *Phytotherapy Research: An International Journal Devoted to Pharmacological and Toxicological Evaluation of Natural Product Derivatives.* 2008 Nov;22(11):1446-9.

[9] Khalaf AA, Al-Aedany AJ, Hussein SF. Activity evaluation of ginger (Zingiberofficinale) alcoholic extract against Candida albicans. In *AIP Conference Proceedings 2020 Dec 4* (Vol. 2290, No. 1, p. 020018). AIP Publishing LLC.

[10] Hassani, M., *Evaluation of antifungal effect of effervescent tablets containing ginger in full dentures with oral fungal infections* (Doctoral dissertation, Tabriz University of Medical Sciences, School of dentistry).2019.

[11] Kandhan TS, Geetha RV. Antimycotic activity of Zingiberofficinale extracts on clinical isolates of Candida albicans. *Drug Invention Today.* 2018 Dec 1;10(12).

[12] Ganeshpurkar A, Thakur A, Jaiswal A. Ginger in Oral Care. *Natural Oral Care in Dental Therapy.* 2020 Jan 30:329-43.

[13] Du Q, Ni S, Guo L, Song W, Zhao K, Liu N, Wang X, Ma X, Fu Y, Tan Q. Effects of Zingiber officinalis (WILLD.) ROSC. Membranes on minor recurrent aphthous stomatitis: a randomized pragmatic trial. *Journal of Traditional Chinese Medical Sciences.* 2018 Jan 1;5(1):58-63.

[14] Haghpanah P, Moghadamnia AA, Zarghami A, Motallebnejad M. Mucobioadhesive containing ginger officinale extract in the management of recurrent aphthous stomatitis: A randomized clinical study. *Caspian Journal of Internal Medicine.* 2015;6(1):3.

[15] Mahyari S, Mahyari B, Emami SA, Malaekeh-Nikouei B, Jahanbakhsh SP, Sahebkar A, Mohammadpour AH. Evaluation of the efficacy of a polyherbal mouthwash containing Zingiberofficinale, Rosmarinus officinalis and Calendula officinalis extracts in patients with gingivitis: A randomized double-blind placebo-controlled trial. *Complementary Therapies in Clinical Practice.* 2016 Feb 1;22:93-8.

[16] Deshpande A, Deshpande N, Raol R, Patel K, Jaiswal V, Wadhwa M. Effect of green tea, ginger plus green tea, and chlorhexidine mouthwash on plaque-induced gingivitis: A randomized clinical trial. *Journal of Indian Society of Periodontology.* 2021 Jul;25(4):307.

[17] Menon P, Perayil J, Fenol A, Peter MR, Lakshmi P, Suresh R. Effectiveness of ginger on pain following periodontal surgery–A randomized cross-over clinical trial. *Journal of Ayurveda and Integrative Medicine.* 2021 Jan 1;12(1):65-9.

[18] Dib K, Ennibi O, Alaoui K, Cherrah Y, Filali-Maltouf A. Antibacterial activity of plant extracts against periodontal pathogens: A systematic review. *Journal of Herbal Medicine.* 2021 Aug 4:100493.

[19] Mardani H, Ghannadi A, Rashnavadi B, Kamali R. The Effect of ginger herbal spray on reducing xerostomia in patients with type II diabetes. *Avicenna journal of phytomedicine.* 2017 Jul;7(4):308.

[20] Dissanayake KG, Waliwita WA, Liyanage RP. A review on medicinal uses of Zingiberofficinale (ginger). *International Journal of Health Sciences and Research.* 2020;10(6).

[21] Rashmi KJ, Tiwari R. Pharmacotherapeutic properties of ginger and its use in diseases of the oral cavity: A narrative review. *Journal of Advanced Oral Research.* 2016 May;7(2):1-6.

[22] Rehman T, Fatima Q. Ginger (Zingiberofficinale): A Mini review. *Int J Complement Alt Med.* 2018;11(2):88-9.

[23] Rynjah D, Chakraborty T, Das A, Islam J, Bordoloi SS, Baishya B, Hasan N. Recent Development in the Formulations of Ginger for Therapeutic Applications and an Overview towards the Action on SARS-COV-2. *International Journal of Pharmaceutical Science and Research*, 2021;12(7):3537-3548.

[24] Sarla GS. Complementary and alternative medicine. *Res Rev J Pharm.* 2019;6(3):1-5p.

[25] Timba PP, Giri SG, Panchal RV. Health benefits and possible Risks of Turmeric, Garlic and Ginger: A short. *Health.* 2019 Apr;6(04):4656-9.

[26] Shooriabi M, Ardakani DS, Mansoori B, Satvati SA, Sharifi R. The effect of ginger extract on radiotherapy-oriented salivation in patients with xerostomia: A double-blind controlled study. *Der Pharmacia Lettre.* 2016;8(15):37-45.

[27] Chamani G, Zarei MR, Mehrabani M, Nakhaee N, Kalaghchi B, Aghili M, Alaee A. Assessment of systemic effects of ginger on salivation in patients with post-radiotherapy xerostomia. *Journal of Oral Health and Oral Epidemiology.* 2017 Jul 5;6(3):130-7.

[28] EL-Sherbiny GM. Antimicrobial susceptibility of bacteria detected from the root canal infection (before and after) root-filled teeth: an in vitro study. *International Journal.* 2015 Jan 1;3(1):4-9.

[29] Valera MC, Oliveira SA, Maekawa LE, Cardoso FG, Chung A, Silva SF, Carvalho CA. Action of Chlorhexidine, Zingiberofficinale, and Calcium Hydroxide on Candida albicans, Enterococcus faecalis, Escherichia coli, and Endotoxin in the root canals. *Journal of Contemporary Dental Practice.* 2016.

[30] Abood FM, Witwit LJ. The Antimicrobial Effect of Some Herbal Extract on Endodontic Infection. *Journal of Pharmaceutical Sciences and Research.* 2018 Jul 1;10(7):1745-7.
[31] Babaeekhou L, Ghane M. Antimicrobial activity of ginger on cariogenic bacteria: Molecular networking and molecular docking analyses. *Journal of Biomolecular Structure and Dynamics.* 2021 Mar 31;39(6):2164-75.
[32] Jain I, Jain P, Bisht D, Sharma A, Srivastava B, Gupta N. Use of traditional Indian plants in the inhibition of caries-causing bacteria-Streptococcus mutans. *Brazilian dental journal.* 2015 Mar; 26:110-5.
[33] Çelik ZC, Yavlal GO, Yanıkoğlu F, Kargul B, Tağtekin D, Stookey GK, Peker S, Hayran O. Do ginger extract, natural honey and bitter chocolate remineralize enamel surface as fluoride toothpastes? An *In vitro* study. *Niger J Clin Pract.* 2021 Sep;24(9):1283-1288. doi: 10.4103/njcp.njcp_683_20.
[34] da Silva TM, Pinheiro CD, Orlandi PP, Pinheiro CC, Pontes GS. Zerumbone from Zingiber zerumbet (L.) smith: a potential prophylactic and therapeutic agent against the cariogenic bacterium Streptococcus mutans. *BMC Complementary and Alternative Medicine.* 2018 Dec;18(1):1-9.
[35] Dentin CL, EGTA E, Tre TH, Cehreli Z, Carvalho C, Steier L, Rossi-fedele G, Kopper PM. The Effect of Zingiberofficinale Roscoe (Ginger) on Dentin Microhardness: An in vitro Study. *Journal of Agricultural Science.* 2017;9(13).
[36] Hassan S, Hafez A, Elbaz MA. Remineralization potential of ginger and rosemary herbals versus sodium fluoride in treatment of white spot lesions: a randomized clinical trial. *Egyptian Dental Journal.* 2021 apr 1;67(2):1677-84.
[37] Attia NM, Ramadan RI. In Vitro Remineralizing Effect of Some Herbals on Initial Enamel Carious Lesions. *Al-Azhar Dental Journal for Girls.* 2021 Apr 1;8(2):325-33.
[38] Ahmed I, Aslam A, Mustafa G, Masood S, Ali MA, Nawaz M. Anti-avian influenza virus H9N2 activity of aqueous extracts of Zingiber officinalis (Ginger) and Allium sativum (Garlic) in chick embryos. *Pak. J. Pharm. Sci.* 2017 Jul;30(4):1341-4.
[39] Schnitzler P, Koch C, Reichling J. Susceptibility of drug-resistant clinical herpes simplex virus type 1 strains to essential oils of ginger, thyme, hyssop, and sandalwood. *Antimicrobial Agents and Chemotherapy.* 2007 May;51(5):1859-62.
[40] Schnitzler P. Essential oils for the treatment of herpes simplex virus infections. *Chemotherapy.* 2019;64(1):1-7.
[41] Lateef FA, Eze BU, Egbunu Z, Jere P, Yusuf D. Evaluation of Some Selected Plant Extracts against Halitosis Causing Organisms. *Journal of Medical and Applied Biosciences.* 10(1):2018.
[42] Senthilkumar V, Ramesh S. Remineralisation Potential of Grape Seed, Ginger Honey-An In vitro Study. *Int J Dentistry Oral Sci.* 2021 Feb 26;8(02):1739-43.
[43] Weidner, M.S. and Sigwart, K., 2000. Investigation of the teratogenic potential of a Zingiberofficinale extract in the rat.*Reproductive Toxicology,15*(1), pp.75-80.

Chapter 3

Image Processing of Ginger Extract via Microwave-Assisted Hydrodistillation

Siti Nuurul Huda Mohammad Azmin[1,*] and Mohd Shukri Mat Nor[2]

[1]Faculty of Agro-Based Industry,
Universiti Malaysia Kelantan Jeli Campus,
Jeli Kelantan, Malaysia
[2]Jeli Agricultural Technology (DC0008911-T),
Kampung Gemang Baru,
Jeli Kelantan, Malaysia

Abstract

Extraction techniques become the primary process to obtain a good quality of plant extraction yield. However, the extraction technique efficiency could be determined by comparing the image processing before and after the extraction process. Image processing of the extract is an important technique to determine the factors affecting the success of the extraction yield. Therefore, this chapter reviews the state-of-the-art development for plant processing and the fundamentals of microwave-assisted hydrodistillation extraction methods. The case study of ginger extraction using microwave-assisted hydrodistillation was demonstrated where the images before and after the extraction processes of ginger were revealed. This chapter also discusses the comparison of the morphological images of the ginger extract.

---

[*] Corresponding Author's Email: huda.ma@umk.edu.my.

In: Ginger and its Health Benefits
Editor: Isla Kermode
ISBN: 978-1-68507-695-5
© 2022 Nova Science Publishers, Inc.

Keywords: extraction technologies, plant processing, natural products, image processing of the extract, microwave assisted-hydrodistillation

Introduction

Ginger has been utilized for a very long time ago as ancient Indians and Chinese have recognized the plant's medicinal properties. They used this plant in curing various health abnormal such as indigestion, diarrhoea, rheumatism, cough, flu and many more. The therapeutic properties of ginger have been stated in the Ayurveda texts of India and ancient Chinese texts. One of the known uses of ginger is its essential oil form known as ginger oil.

Essential oils are the volatile, organic constituents of secondary metabolites produced by odoriferous or fragrant plant matter, contributing to fragrance and flavour. These oils are necessary because they were thought to be crucial to the plant's life processes or represent the various essence of taste and odour since they carry the plant's meaning. The oils evaporate when they are exposed to the air and thus, is capable of distillation or obtained from plant material through various volatility extraction methods. The oils' characteristics differ from fixed oils (fatty oil) extracted from the seed, contain a low odour, and are non-volatile.

The aroma and flavour of ginger come from its essential oil, usually known as ginger oil. Previous studies found that there is more than 200 different volatiles have been identified in ginger oil. Some researchers identified that ginger contains up to 3% essential oil, with sesquiterpenoids and zingiberene as the main constituents. On the other hand, smaller amounts of other sesquiterpenoids (β-sesquiphellandrene, bisabolene and farnesene) and a small monoterpenoid fraction (β-phellandrene, cineol, and citral) are also found. Typical ginger oil has been characterized by many sesquiterpene hydrocarbons (zingiberene, ar-curcumene, á-bisabolene, and á-sesquiphellandrene), while essential monoterpenoids usually include geranial, neral and camphene (Martins et al. 2001; B M Lawrence 2000). Even though these compounds are characterized as typical ginger oils, the literature presents that ginger oil composition is highly variable (Gurib-Fakim et al. 2002; B M Lawrence 2000). The composition of ginger oil is influenced by a few factors such as geographical origin, the freshness of the ginger rhizome, drying process and temperature used, the harvest seasons, method of harvest and analytical methodology that might contribute to the disparity of published ginger oil analyses.

The odour of ginger could not be characterized by one particular compound but rather by a mixture of various terpenoids and some non-terpenoids. It has been considered unlikely that the typical aroma of ginger would ever be utterly unrevealed due to the enormous complexity of the oil. The ginger aroma profile and the composition of the volatile compounds have been differently reported, depending on the harvested place (British Pharmacopoeia, Volume, and II 2004; COUNCIL 2004; China 2000). Many studies related to food processing and distribution have reported the influence on the composition of volatile compounds by the extraction process, irradiation, cooking dan drying of ginger (Lien et al. 2003; Willetts, Ekangaki, and Eden 2003; Smith et al. 2004).

Microwave Assisted-Hydrodistillation

Microwave assisted-hydrodistillation is an advanced hydrodistillation method based on a microwave oven and performed at atmospheric pressure. The principle of this method is based on the 'molecular friction' or dielectric loss. The material molecules become stimulated and rotate a million times for a second in response to the electromagnetic field. The quick rotations generate heat in the material in a similar manner to friction.

The selected matrix must compose dipolar or ionic species to ensure that the microwave irradiation generates heat when interacting with the matrix. The dipoles or ions are induced to move the matrix by the interaction of the applied irradiation. In receptive materials, polar molecules and free ions respond to these fields by creating molecular friction, resulting in heat throughout the material mass. For example, water is an electric dipole with a positive charge at one end and a negative charge at another. Thus, the dipole molecule undergoes oscillations in response to the high frequency of the field's polarity changes as it tries to align itself by an alternating electric field of the microwaves. This molecular movement produces high-frequency energy absorbed before transforming into thermal energy as the rotating molecules hit other molecules and put them into an intermolecular friction motion. Figure 1 presents the experimental apparatus set up using microwave assisted-hydrodistillation.

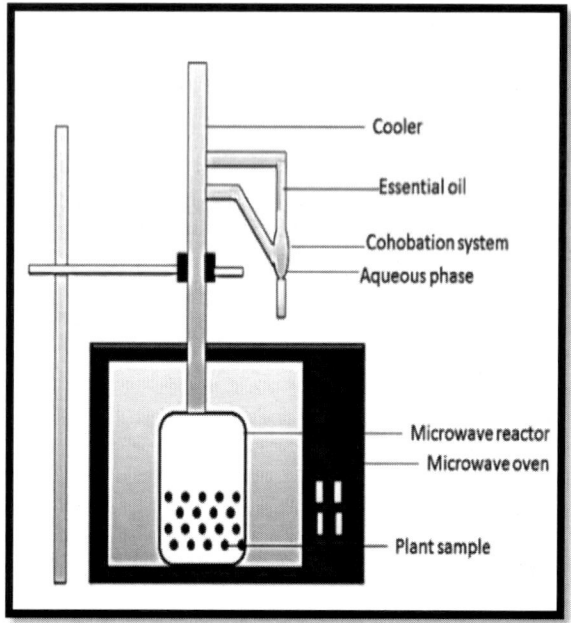

Figure 1. Microwave equipment assisted hydrodistillation extraction.

Advantages of Microwave Assisted-Hydrodistillation

The extraction method using microwave assisted-hydrodistillation offers rapid processing, which highly accelerates the extraction process without causing considerable changes in the volatile oil composition. The phenomenon has been elaborated by Paré and Bélanger (1997). The obtained yield by the two methods is the same order of magnitude, but the observed extraction time is different. The efficiency of microwave assisted-hydrodistillation strongly depends on the dielectric constant of water and the matrix (Brachet, Christen, and Veuthey 2002; Azmin et al. 2016). It gives a meaning that the rapid delivery of energy to the total volume of solvent or sample is caused by microwave assisted-hydrodistillation leads to a rapid rise in the temperature. In the form of dielectric heating, microwave heating is the generation of heat in materials of low electrical conductivity by applying a high-frequency electric field. Due to its efficient volumetric heat production, microwave energy is a superior alternative to several thermal applications, as shown in Table 1.

Table 1. Comparison of conversion efficiencies between various heating sources

Appliance	Temp, °C	Appliance rating, W	Time, min	Energy used, kWh	Energy cost, US$
Electric oven	177	2000	60	2	0.17
Convection oven	163	1853	45	1.39	0.12
Gas oven	177	36	60	3.57	0.07
Frying pan	216	900	60	0.9	0.07
Toaster oven	218	1140	50	0.95	0.08
Crockpot	93	100	420	0.7	0.06
Microwave oven	High	1440	15	0.36	0.03

Disadvantages of Microwave Assisted-Hydrodistillation

The extraction of essential oils is obtained by introducing the plant sample in a multi-mode microwave cavity. The size and shape of the vessel are crucial since the vessel volume is charged with the batch as it depends on the cavity dimension of the microwave brand. According to the previous research, the needed volume ranging from one to two litres. Another disadvantage of microwave assisted-hydrodistillation is the vessel or reactor must be made from non-metallic, and metal sensors or other devices made from metal are avoided. The glassware components applied in this method, such as reflux condenser, a stirring bar, a water cooling bath or a metal probe, must be directly connected to the reactor and placed outside the oven. As a safety regulation, direct visual and manual access to the reactor is forbidden to the operator.

Besides, the non-uniformity property of microwave assisted-hydrodistillation is one of the method drawbacks. The uniformity is a function of material characteristics. These cavity boundary conditions affect the field penetration depth, thermal runaway, high field age effects, micro-arcing and high displacement of current around contact point between particular loads. These factors determine the possible modes that might be excited inside the cavity, which superimpose to create an uneven distribution field within the cavity. The phenomenon can cause the temperature result to be non-uniformity. There are some techniques to improve the heating uniformity, such as using rotary deflector plates to excite different modes and change the cavities boundary conditions (providing a continuous moving field environment), increasing cavity size (increasing the number of modes and hence improving the field uniformity), moving the material to be heated (the most common way of overcoming non-uniform heating and the most effective when liquids are concerned) and modulate the magnetron frequency (altering the amount of power coupled to various modes),

Image Processing of Plant Extract Using Scanning Electron Microscopy

Solid-liquid extraction of plant materials is the most common method to obtain either essential oil or crude extract. In comparing the efficiency of the solid-liquid extraction method, scanning electron microscopy could be utilized as one of the analyzed methods. Scanning electron microscopy equipment has been widely applied to observe the morphological image of any samples, including plants. Typically, the studied plant image will be compared at two stages which are before and after treating the samples. The comparison is conducted either to identify the changes of a plant cell, prove that the completion of the extraction process occurred, or compare the glandular modifications concerning different methods and extraction time used. Thus, this chapter will use the extraction of ginger using microwave-assisted hydrodistillation as a case study.

Case Study

Ginger has been used as a spice for over 2000 years (Bartley and Jacobs 2000). It also has been applied as a medicine since ancient times, as recorded in early Sanskrit and Chinese texts and ancient Greek, Roman and Arabic medical pieces of literature (Bone et al. 1990). In traditional Indian medicine or Ayurveda, ginger and many other spices have been used as medicine (Langer 1998). The fresh and dried ginger rhizomes have been practised worldwide as a spice, while ginger extract has been extensively consumed in food, beverages, and confectionery industries. Ginger oil contains a high content of sesquiterpene hydrocarbon (including zingiberene, ar-curcumene, and âbisabolene and á-sesquiphellandrene) and important monoterpenoids (such as geranial, neral and camphene) (Brian M Lawrence 2011). The variable of the composition of ginger oil is influenced by several factors such as geographical origin, the freshness of the ginger rhizome, drying process and temperature, method of harvest and analytical methodology. Thus, the objective of this case study is to compare the glandular change in the ginger extract. Morphological images of dried ginger and ginger after the extraction process were observed. Microwave-assisted hydrodistillation extraction was applied as an extraction method of ginger oil. Noted that, this case study focuses on the morphological image of the plant sample instead of the extraction yield of extract.

The case study will focus on the extraction of ginger with its morphological image before and after extraction processes. The procedure composes of three different parts, which are plant material preparation, drying and extraction process.

Preparation of plant material started with the longitudinally slicing of ginger rhizomes with 1 mm of average thickness. The sliced ginger then was under-shade dried until the dryness percentage achieving to 30%. The dryness percentage was computed using Equation 1:

$$Dryness\ (\%) = \frac{W_0 - W_f}{W_0} X\ 100 \qquad \text{(Equation 1)}$$

where W_0 is the initial weight of ginger and W_f is the final weight of ginger.

The 30% dryness of ginger then was ground and sealed in the desiccator to avoid any fungal activities before it was used in the extraction. The dried ginger was also tested for its morphological image.

The microwave-assisted hydrodistillation extraction method was used to extract the essential oil of ginger. The involved apparatus is shown in Figure 1. In this case study, water was applied as an extraction solvent to extract the essential oil from the ginger sample. The extraction time was fixed to one hour while the ratio of ginger to water was 1:8. After one hour of the extraction process, the mixture of ginger and water was filtered using Whatman filter paper number 1. The residue then was dried before it was tested for the morphological image. The glandular image of the ginger sample before and after the extraction process was compared.

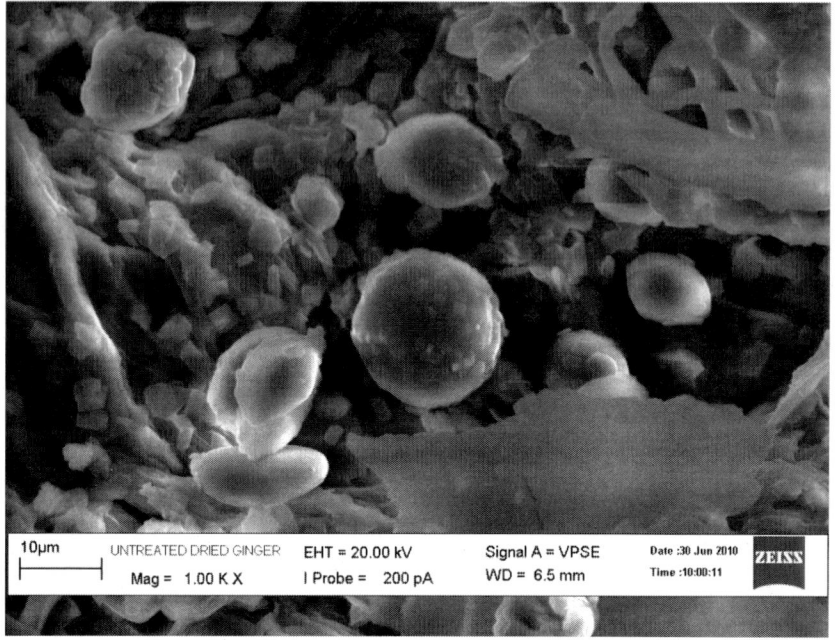

Figure 2. Micrograph of the untreated gland ginger before the extraction at 1000 X magnification.

Image of Dried Ginger Sample

Figure 2 shows the micrograph of the glandular structure of dried ginger before the extraction process at 1000 X magnification. The image of the dried ginger was observed under the scanning electron microscopy (SEM) model Carl Zeiss, ZEISS EVO 50. This SEM model equips with 2.0 to 4.5 nm resolution at 30 kV, an acceleration voltage of 0.2 to 30 kV, and magnification on 5 to 1, 000, 000. This scanning electron microscopy can handle 250 mm of specimen diameter at the analytical working distance of 8.5 mm owing to the combination of the large movement stage, inclined detectors, and conical objective lens.

Image of Ginger after the Extraction Process

Figure 3 shows the micrograph of the glandular structure of ginger after 1 hour of microwave-assisted hydrodistillation extraction at 700 X magnification. In this figure, most of the glandular structure appeared disrupted entirely. The observation of the ginger glandular after extraction procedure also used the same brand and model of scanning electron microscopy for the dried ginger sample.

Comparison of a Morphological Image of Plant Extract

Essential oil plays a vital role for human beings as it is valuable because of its medicinal and fragrant properties. The essential oil has been widely applied in the pharmaceutical and cosmetic industries. Therefore, the localization of the oil in the plant attracts the researcher's attention. It has been proven that the glandular structures of the plant are the primary sites of the secretion and storage of essential oil in certain plant species (Ringer, Davis, and Croteau 2005; Sharma, Sangwan, and Sangwan 2003). Essential oil is located in well-defined secretory structures such as oil cells, glandular trichomes, oil or resin ducts or glandular epidermis (Craker and Simon 1992). These glands usually develop on the surface of leaves, bracts, petals, and other organs of aromatic herbs. During the maturity stage of the leaves or stem, the oil is stored in the subcuticular space that is formed at the gland apex. However, the mechanism of oil released from matured glands has not been published yet, and the conflicting views on the oil released were expressed between researchers. Bosabalidis and Tsekos (1984) mentioned the rupture of the cuticle at the later stages of secretion, while Werker et al., (1985) reported that the secretion material of the plant (*Labiatae*) was not released unless some external factors damaged the gland. The extraction rate of essential oil is often controlled by intraparticle resistances of the herbaceous matrices, which arise from the location of the essential oil within the aromatic herbs (Bartle et al. 1990).

Figures 2 and 3 present a significantly different glandular structure of ginger plant material before and after the extraction. The gland structure after the extraction of ginger shows that the glandular was completely ruptured. One hour of extraction time is sufficient to destroy the glandular structures. It is because the aid of microwave reduces the extraction time of essential oil. The observation of this case study found that the microwave treatment affected the cell structure due to the sudden temperature rise and increased internal pressure. The phenomenon occurred as the targeted heating of the free water molecules in the gland and vascular systems, leading to localized heating causing dramatic expansion, with subsequent ruptures of their cell walls (García-Ayuso et al. 2000). Rupture of gland cell wall permits the ginger oil to flow towards the water solvent. The microwave-assisted hydrodistillation extraction method utilizes three ways of heat transfer (irradiation, conduction and convection) within the sample which contributes to the fast heat produced within the glands and from outside of the glands (Ferhat et al. 2006).

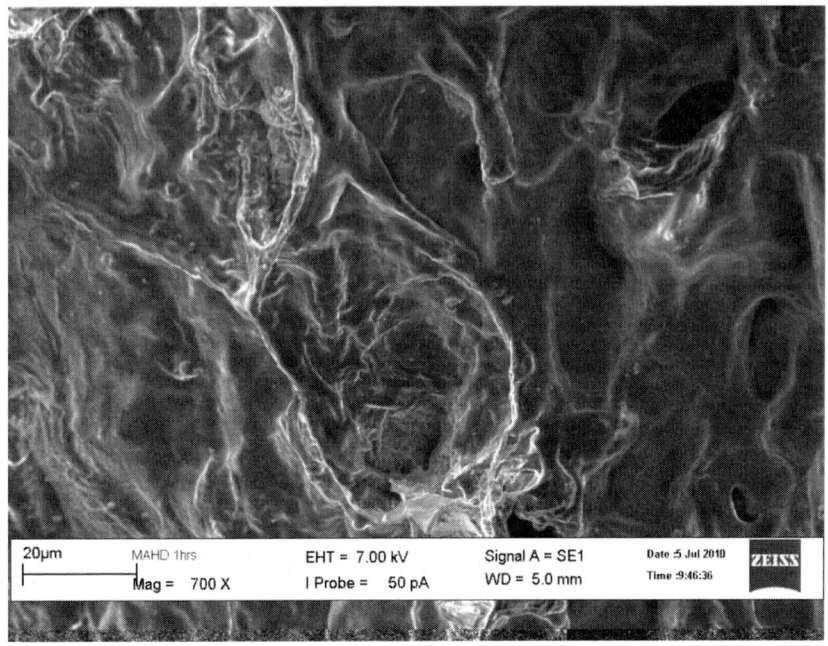

Figure 3. Micrograph of the glandular structure of ginger after 1 hour of microwave-assisted hydrodistillation extraction at 700 X magnification.

The Relation between Image Processing and Extraction Yield for Plants

This case study extracted dried ginger using the microwave assisted-hydrodistillation method to measure the extraction yield. Three power levels (200 W, 225 W and 275 W) were applied to study the effect of microwave power on the extraction yield at various extraction times. The ratio of ginger to water was 1:8, while the ginger dryness was 90%. It means that the ginger is to be extracted composing of 10% water only. As depicted in Figure 4, the highest ginger oil yield (1.796%) was obtained by 200 W power of microwave for 90 minutes. After 90 minutes, the extraction yield becomes constant, meaning that there is no more ginger oil to be extracted from the dried ginger.

Some reported investigations revealed that microwave-assisted hydrodistillation could save energy and time. For example, Golmakani and Rezaei (2008) reported that this method could extract the full recovery of essential oil from *Thymus vulgaris* L. within two hours operation while four hours for complete recovery of essential oil using hydrodistillation method. The results presented that the performance of microwave assisted-hydrodistillation is 50% better than the hydrodistillation method. The microwave-assisted-hydrodistillation process needed a shorter extraction time compared to the conventional hydrodistillation method. This is due to the more efficient heat flow involved using the microwave, which applies high-frequency and is very short of radio waves. However, the classic conductive heating methods do not heat the entire plant sample but only heat the plant's surface (Kaufmann and Christen 2002). The movement of the microwaves through the sample generates internal heat and at the surface of the treated plant material. In addition, as the conventional hydrodistillation method applies heat only on the material's surface, the temperature must not be too high to avoid burning. This traditional method contributes to extend the extraction time to the thermal conductivity of the fluids. Comparatively, the percentage yield of ginger oil conducted by Onyenekwe and Hashimoto (1999) from Nigeria ginger using hydrodistillation method was 2.4% (w/w). These discrepancies may be explained by variety, soil, locality and climate conditions (Baydar, Baydar, and Debener 2004).

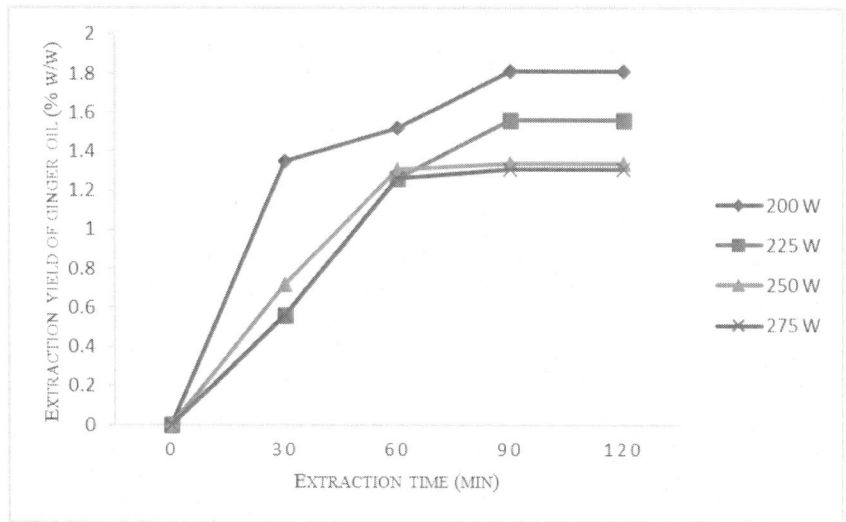

Figure 4. Effect of extraction time at a different power level of the microwave assisted-hydrodistillation extraction method.

On the other hand, the difference in microwave power level also affects ginger oil's percentage yield. For instance, at a microwave power of 275 W, the extraction achieved the highest result, faster than 250 W, 225 W and 200 W. This result is supported by their induction time (time needed to reach the extraction temperature), where 275 W was recorded as the fastest time than others which only requires 18 minutes. The rests were 21 minutes for 250 W, 24 minutes for 225 W and 27 minutes for 200 W. The induction time is parallel to the extraction yield, where 275 W gave the highest extraction yield of ginger oil. Observing the micrograph of ginger's glandular structure is ruptured as the longer extraction time is conducted, as shown in Figure 4.

Improvement for the Developed Research in Image Processing for Plants

Essential oil production and processing have gained serious consideration either from practical or fundamental aspects by industries and researchers for the last few decades. One of the focuses in developing an effective extraction method is to reduce the extraction time in essential oil production. Selecting the best solid-liquid extraction method would improve the oil quality and reduce energy and operating costs.

Image processing for plants could help to enhance the solid-liquid extraction yield by determining the best method that can easily rupture the cell wall. Thus, the optimum conditions could be selected based on the morphological image, where the correlation of extraction yield with the images can be the evidence.

Conclusion

The morphological image of ginger has been revealed in the case study. The micrograph images of the glandular structure for ginger were compared for two conditions: before and after the extraction processes. The result showed that the ruptures of the glandular system occurred. It gives a meaning that the essential oil from ginger could be extracted via microwave-assisted hydrodistillation technique. The efficiency of the extraction method to get the ginger oil is vitally important as this oil could be beneficial to human health.

Acknowledgment

This study was financially supported by the Ministry of Education Malaysia, Fundamental Research Grant Scheme for Research Acculturation of Early Career Researchers (FRGS-RACER, R/FRGS/A0700/01552A/003/2019/00665) and Universiti Malaysia Kelantan, UMK Prototype Research Grant (UMK-PRO 2020, R/PRO/A0700/01552A/004/2020/00872). These supports are gratefully acknowledged.

References

Azmin, Siti Nuurul Huda Mohammad, Zainuddin Abdul Manan, Sharifah Rafidah Wan Alwi, Lee Suan Chua, Azizul Azri Mustaffa. & Nor Alafiza Yunus. (2016). "Herbal Processing and Extraction Technologies." *Separation and Purification Reviews, 45* (4), 305–20. https://doi.org/10.1080/15422119.2016.1145395.
Bartle, Keith D., Anthony A Clifford, Steven B Hawthorne, John J Langenfeld, David J Miller. & Robert Robinson. (1990). "A Model for Dynamic Extraction Using a Supercritical Fluid." *The Journal of Supercritical Fluids, 3* (3), 143–49.
Bartley, John P. & Amanda L Jacobs. (2000). "Effects of Drying on Flavour Compounds in Australian-grown Ginger (Zingiber Officinale)." *Journal of the Science of Food and Agriculture, 80* (2), 209–15.
Baydar, Nilgün Göktürk, Hasan Baydar. & Thomas Debener. (2004). "Analysis of Genetic Relationships among Rosa Damascena Plants Grown in Turkey by Using AFLP and Microsatellite Markers." *Journal of Biotechnology, 111* (3), 263–67.
Bone, M. E., Wilkinson, D. J., Young, J. R., McNeil, J. & Charlton, S. (1990). "Ginger Root—a New Antiemetic The Effect of Ginger Root on Postoperative Nausea and Vomiting after Major Gynaecological Surgery." *Anaesthesia, 45* (8), 669–71.
Bosabalidis, A. M. & Tsekos, I. (1984). "Glandular Hair Formation in Origanum Species." *Annals of Botany, 53* (4), 559–63.
Brachet, Anne, Philippe Christen. & Veuthey, J. L. (2002). "Focused Microwave-assisted Extraction of Cocaine and Benzoylecgonine from Coca Leaves." *Phytochemical Analysis: An International Journal of Plant Chemical and Biochemical Techniques, 13* (3), 162–69.
British Pharmacopoeia, CDROM, I Volume, and Monographs II. (2004). "Medicinal and Pharmaceutical Substances." Stationary Office, London.
China, Pharmacopoeia Commission. (2000). *Pharmacopoeia of the People's Republic of China.* Chemical Industry Press.
COUNCIL, OF EUROPE. (2004). "European Pharmacopoeia 5.0." *Council of Europe.*
Craker, Lyle E. & James E Simon. (1992). *Herbs, Spices, and Medicinal Plants: Recent Advances in Botany, Horticulture, and Pharmacology.,* Vol. *1.* Psychology Press.

Ferhat, Mohamed A., Brahim Y Meklati, Jacqueline Smadja. & Farid Chemat. (2006). "An Improved Microwave Clevenger Apparatus for Distillation of Essential Oils from Orange Peel." *Journal of Chromatography A*, *1112* (1–2), 121–26.

García-Ayuso, L. E., Velasco, J., Dobarganes, M. C. & Luque De Castro, M. D. (2000). "Determination of the Oil Content of Seeds by Focused Microwave-Assisted Soxhlet Extraction." *Chromatographia*, *52* (1–2), 103–8.

Golmakani, Mohammad-Taghi. & Karamatollah Rezaei. (2008). "Comparison of Microwave-Assisted Hydrodistillation Withthe Traditional Hydrodistillation Method in the Extractionof Essential Oils from Thymus Vulgaris L." *Food Chemistry*, *109* (4), 925–30.

Gurib-Fakim, Ameenah, Naheeda Maudarbaccus, David Leach, Luigino Doimo. & Hans Wohlmuth. (2002). "Essential Oil Composition of Zingiberaceae Species from Mauritius." *Journal of Essential Oil Research*, *14* (4), 271–73.

Kaufmann, Béatrice. & Philippe Christen. (2002). "Recent Extraction Techniques for Natural Products: Microwave-assisted Extraction and Pressurised Solvent Extraction." *Phytochemical Analysis: An International Journal of Plant Chemical and Biochemical Techniques*, *13* (2), 105–13.

Langer, Robert. (1998). "Drug Delivery and Targeting." *Nature*, *392* (6679 Suppl), 5–10.

Lawrence, B M. (2000). "Ginger Oil in Progress in Essential Oils." *Perfumer & Flavorist*, *25*, 46–57.

Lawrence, Brian M. (2011). "Progress in Essential Oils." *Perfumer & Flavorist*, *36* (11), 52–58.

Lien, Han-Chung, Wei Ming Sun, Yen-Hsueh Chen, Hyerang Kim, William Hasler. & Chung Owyang. (2003). "Effects of Ginger on Motion Sickness and Gastric Slow-Wave Dysrhythmias Induced by Circular Vection." *American Journal of Physiology-Gastrointestinal and Liver Physiology*, *284* (3), G481–89.

Martins, A. P., Salgueiro, L., Goncalves, M. J., Proençada Cunha, A., Vila, R., Canigueral, S., Mazzoni, V., Tomi, F. & Casanova, J. (2001). "Essential Oil Composition and Antimicrobial Activity of Three Zingiberaceae from S. Tome e Principe." *Planta Medica*, *67* (06), 580–84.

Onyenekwe, Paul Chidozie. & Seiji Hashimoto. (1999). "The Composition of the Essential Oil of Dried Nigerian Ginger (Zingiber Officinale Roscoe)." *European Food Research and Technology*, *209* (6), 407–10.

Paré, J. R. J. & Bélanger, J. M. R. (1997). *Instrumental Methods in Food Analysis*. Elsevier.

Ringer, Kerry L., Edward M Davis. & Rodney Croteau. (2005). "Monoterpene Metabolism. Cloning, Expression, and Characterization of (−)-Isopiperitenol/(−)-Carveol Dehydrogenase of Peppermint and Spearmint." *Plant Physiology*, *137* (3), 863–72.

Sharma, Shruti., Sangwan, N. S. & Rajender S Sangwan. (2003). "Developmental Process of Essential Oil Glandular Trichome Collapsing in Menthol Mint." *Current Science*, 544–50.

Smith, Caroline, Caroline Crowther, Kristyn Willson, Neil Hotham. & Vicki McMillian. (2004). "A Randomized Controlled Trial of Ginger to Treat Nausea and Vomiting in Pregnancy." *Obstetrics & Gynecology*, *103* (4), 639–45.

Werker, Ella., Ravid, U. & Putievsky, E. (1985). "Structure of Glandular Hairs and Identification of the Main Components of Their Secreted Material in Some Species of the Labiatae." *Israel Journal of Plant Sciences, 34* (1), 31–45.

Willetts, Karen E., Abie Ekangaki. & John A Eden. (2003). "Effect of a Ginger Extract on Pregnancy-induced Nausea: A Randomised Controlled Trial." *Australian and New Zealand Journal of Obstetrics and Gynaecology, 43* (2), 139–44.

Biographical Sketch

Name: Siti Nuurul Huda, Mohammad Azmin
Affiliation: Universiti Malaysia Kelantan
Education: PhD in Chemical Engineering
Business Address: Faculty of Agro-based Industry, Universiti Malaysia Kelantan Jeli Campus, 17600 Jeli Kelantan.
Research and Professional Experience: 5 years plus in research and teaching.
Professional Appointments: Senior lecturer.
Honors: Ts. Dr.
Publications from the Last 3 Years:
Books and book chapter

[1] **Siti Nuurul Huda Mohammad Azmin** et al., (2021*). Mulberry leaf: The story of potential miracle plant*. UPSI publisher. (will be published on October 2021).

[2] **Siti Nuurul Huda Mohammad Azmin.** (2021). *Physico-chemical Properties of Mulberry Leaf. Mulberry leaf: The story of potential miracle plant.* UPSI publisher. (will be published on October 2021).

[3] **Siti Nuurul Huda Mohammad Azmin.** & Huck Ywih Ch'ng. (2020). Curry Leaf (Murraya koenigii): *The story of potential Miracle Plant.* Beau Bassin: Mauritius. LAP LAMBERT Academic Publishing (ISBN: 978-620-0-50574-3). pp. 0-57.

[4] **Siti Nuurul Huda Mohammad Azmin.** (2020). Physico-chemical Properties of Curry Leaf. Curry leaf (Murayya koenigii): *The story of potential miracle plant,* Beau Bassin: Mauritius. LAP LAMBERT Academic Publishing (ISBN: 978-620-0-50574-3), 26-30.

[5] Abduralınan Hamid Nour, Azhari Hamid Nour. & **Siti Nuurul Huda Mohammad Azmin.** (2010). *Pipeline Transportation for Heavy Crude*

Oil via Oil-in-Water Emulsions. LAP Lambert Academic Publishing (2011-07-03), ISBN-13: 978-3845400303; ISBN-10: 3845400307.

Journals

[1] **Siti Nuurul Huda Mohammad Azmin**, Nur Solehin Sulaiman, Mohd Shukri Mat Nor. & Ade Chandra Iwansyah. (2021). A Review on Recent Advances on Natural Plant Pigments in Foods: Functions, Extraction, Importance and Challenges. Under review in *Journal of Food Reviews International*.

[2] **Siti Nuurul Huda Mohammad Azmin**, Nur Solehin Sulaiman, Mohd Shukri Mat Nor. & Palsan Sannasi Abdullah. (2021). Evaluation of Moisturising Lip Balm Comprise of Natural Pigment from Tomato. In Press.

[3] **Siti Nuurul Huda Mohammad Azmin**. & Mohd Shukri Mat Nor. (2021). Optimization of formulation conditions for anti-wrinkle and whitening peel-off face mask from banana peels and mulberry leaves extracts using response surface methodology. In Press.

[4] **Siti Nuurul Huda Mohammad Azmin**. & Mohd Shukri Mat Nor. (2021). Processing and Characterization of Bioplastic Film Fabricated from a hybrid of Cocoa Pod Husk and Kenaf for the Application in Food Industries. *Under Review in the British Food Journal*.

[5] **Siti Nuurul Huda Mohammad Azmin**, Aina Sofea Abdul Halim. & Mohd Shukri Mat Nor. (2021). Physicochemical analysis of natural herbal medicated ointment enriched with Cymbopogon nardus and virgin coconut oil. In *IOP Conference Series: Earth and Environmental Science*, (Vol. 765, No. 1, p. 012040). IOP Publishing.

[6] **Siti Nuurul Huda Mohammad Azmin**. & Mohd Shukri Mat Nor. (2021). Property model prediction of the boiling point for pure and mixture solvents applied in herbal extraction. In *IOP Conference Series: Earth and Environmental Science*, (Vol. 765, No. 1, p. 012100). IOP Publishing.

[7] **Siti Nuurul Huda Mohammad Azmin**, Nurul Aqilah Yosri, Nur Solehin Sulaiman, Mohd Shukri Mat Nor. & Palsan Sannasi Abdullah. (2021). "Stability Analysis of Moisturising Lip Balm using Natural

Pigment from Daucus carota" *Chemical Engineering Transaction*, (83), 49-54.

[8] Gunavathy Selvarajh, Ch'ng Huck Ywih, Norhafizah Md Zain, Palsan Sannasi Abdullah. & **Siti Nuurul Huda Mohammad Azmin.** (2021). "Improving Soil Nitrogen Availability and Rice Growth Performance on a Tropical Acid Soil via Mixture of Rice Husk and Rice Straw Biochars." *Applied Sciences*, 11, no. 1, (2021), 108.

[9] Huda Awang, Jayanthi, Zul Ariff Abdul Latiff, Leony Tham Yew Seng, **Siti Nuurul Huda Mohammad Azmin.** & Palsan Sannasi Abdullah. (2020). "Optimization and Modelling of the Removal of Groundwater Turbidity by Nanomagnetic Adsorbent Composite". *IOP Conference Series: Earth and Environmental Science*, vol. 596, no. 1, p. 012047. IOP Publishing.

[10] **Siti Nuurul Huda Mohammad Azmin**, Aisha Amira Abd Razak. & Mohd Shukri Mat Nor. (2020). "Physicochemical Analysis of Medicated Ointment Enriched with Ginger (*Zingiber officinale*) Oil." *IOP Conference Series: Earth and Environmental Science.*, Vol. 596. No. 1. IOP Publishing.

[11] **Siti Nuurul Huda Mohammad Azmin.** & Mohd Shukri Mat Nor. (2020). Chemical Fingerprint of Centella Asiatica's Bioactive Compounds in The Ethanolic and Aqueous Extracts. *Journal of advances in Biomarker Sciences and Technology*, 2, 35-44.

[12] **Siti Nuurul Huda Mohammad Azmin**, Najah Aliah binti Mohd Hayat. & Mohd Shukri Mat Nor. (2020). Development and characterization of food packaging bioplastic film from cocoa pod husk cellulose incorporated with sugarcane bagasse fibre. *Journal of Bioresources and Bioproducts*, 5(4), 259-266.

[13] **Siti Nuurul Huda Mohammad Azmin**, Nurul Aqilah Yosri, Nur Solehin Sulaiman, Mohd Shukri Mat Nor. & Palsan Sannasi Abdullah. (2020). "Sensory Evaluation of Appearance and Texture of Carrot Lip Balms Containing Virgin Coconut Oil." In *IOP Conference Series: Earth and Environmental Science*, vol. 549, no. 1, p. 012071. IOP Publishing.

[14] **Siti Nuurul Huda Mohammad Azmin**, Nurshafieera Idayu Mat Jaine. & Mohd Shukri Mat Nor. (2020). "Physicochemical and sensory

evaluations of moisturising lip balm using natural pigment from Beta vulgaris." *Cogent Engineering, 7.01*, 1788297.

[15] Mohd Rifin, N. F., Mat Nor, M. S. & **Mohammad Azmin, S. N. H.** (2019). Antioxidant Activity of Salacca zalacca and Eleiodoxa conferta Fruits Skin. *International conference of Asean Food, 19.*

Chapter 4

Effects of Ginger (*Zingiber officinale* Roscoe 1807) on Health Promotion

Karina Zanoti Fonseca[1,*], PhD, Ferlando Lima Santos[1,†], PhD and Franceli da Silva[2,‡], PhD

[1]Nutritionist, Federal University of Recôncavo da Bahia,
Center for Health Sciences, Santo Antônio de Jesus, Bahia, Brazil
[2]Agricultural Engineer, Federal University of Recôncavo da Bahia, Centro de Ciências Exatas, Ambientais e Biológicas/CCAAB,
Cruz das Almas, Bahia, Brazil

Abstract

Ginger (*Zingiber officinale* Roscoe 1807) is a perennial monocot rhizome of the family Zingiberaceae native from southeast Asia. It is widely used worldwide as spice and as beverage flavor, mainly in Asian products. Ginger is not only used as food, but also in the traditional Asian medicine. Several studies have focused on the health benefits of ginger consumption based on the fact that India and China have been traditionally using it to treat asthma, headache, infectious diseases, rheumatoid arthritis and helminthiasis. Its main effects are related to its anti-inflammatory, anti-tumor, anti-hyperglycemic and anti-lipidemic activities. One of its bioactive compounds, gingerol, prevents hyperlipidemia induced by lipid-rich diets by regulating the expression

---

[*] Corresponding Author's Email: karinaufrb@ufrb.edu.br.
[†] Corresponding Author's Email: ferlando@ufrb.edu.br.
[‡] Corresponding Author's Email: franceli@ufrb.edu.br.

In: Ginger and its Health Benefits
Editor: Isla Kermode
ISBN: 978-1-68507-695-5
© 2022 Nova Science Publishers, Inc.

of enzymes involved in cholesterol homeostasis. Ginger is considered a safe and effective antidiabetic adjuvant and shows beneficial effects on lipid profile, insulin resistance and weight loss. Its protective effects against cancer are among its most studied properties and are related to the induction of tumor cell apoptosis and inhibition of cell proliferation. This chapter addresses the state of the art of research on the use of ginger in health promotion.

Keywords: health, spice, *Zingiberaceae*, disease prevention

Introduction

Ginger (*Zingiber officinale Roscoe* 1807) is a perennial monocot rhizome of the family Zingiberaceae native from south-east Asia (Si et al., 2018). The Zingiberaceaea family includes species such as turmeric and cardamom (Ujang et al., 2015). Its cultivation originated with the Austronesian people and was transferred to other regions through the Indo-pacific about 5,000 years ago (Ravindran e Babu, 2016).

The spice had a religious meaning among the Austronesian, who used it in healing and spiritual protection rituals and ship-blessing ceremonies. Ginger was introduced to India during the Austronesian expansion and then transported to Middle East and the Mediterranean by traders around the first century (Ujang et al., 2015). The plant has also been used by ancient Romans and Greeks and is considered the first spice to be exported from Asia to Europe (Christenhusz e Byng, 2016).

Ginger is widely used worldwide as spice and beverage flavor, mainly in Asian products. Due to its pungent and spicy flavor, its abundance, low cost of cultivation and consumption safety, its use has increased in the last decades (SRINIVASAN, 2017).

Taxonomic classification (USDA, 2021):

- Kingdom: *Plantae*
- Phylum: *Magnoliophyta*
- Class: *Liliopsida*
- Order: *Zingiberales*
- Family: *Zingiberaceae*
- Genus: *Zingiber* p. Moller, 1754
- Species: *Zingiber officinale* Roscoe, 1807.

Ginger is used not only as food but also in the Traditional Eastern Medicine (Ali et al., 2008).

The health benefits of ginger consumption have been the focus of several studies, based on the fact that India and China have traditionally used it to treat asthma, headache (Ali et al., 2008; Li et al., 2019), infectious diseases, rheumatoid arthritis and helminthiasis (Ali et al., 2008).

On present days, ginger is used to treat gastrointestinal ulcers, cancer, arthritis and vomit (Idris et al., 2019, Getaneh, Guadie e Tefera, 2021).

The main health-promoting effects of ginger are related to its antiinflammatory, anti-tumor, anti-hyperglycemic and anti-lipidemic activities (Srinivasan, 2017). Its active compounds may vary according to the place of cultivation and rhizome status (*in natura* or dried) (Sang et al., 2020). Based on this, Li et al., (2019) have considered that ginger has a promising role on health promotion.

Ginger has several active compounds, including oil resin, terpenes, zingerone, paradols, vitamins, minerals, gingerols and shogaols (Teng et al., 2019). The main bioactive compounds with pharmacological importance are the gingerols (Ghafoor et al., 2020) and shogaols, non-volatile pungent compounds (Mao et al., 2019).

The objective of this chapter is to provide a systematic review of the literature on the health-promoting properties of ginger (*Zingiber officinale* Roscoe).

Health-Promoting Properties

Hypolipemiant Properties

Ginger is known to stimulate digestion by increasing pancreatic lipase activity and secretion of bile salts (Prakash and Srinivasan, 2012), being effective in suppressing cholesterol and lipid build-up.

One of ginger's bioactive compounds, gingerol, prevents hyperlipidemia induced by lipid-rich diets, regulating the expression of enzymes involved in cholesterol homeostasis (Srinivasan, 2017).

Low doses of ginger, around 2g/day, were capable of reducing triglyceride and LDL levels of adult subjects. Doses above 2g/day, supplemented on intervals of less than 50 days, resulted in a positive total hypolipemiant effect. Along with this effect, favorable results were observed on HDL levels (Jafarnejad et al., 2017).

Anti-Diabetic Properties

The incidence of diabetes mellitus is high and is increasing globally mainly due to the prevalence of obesity and unhealthy lifestyles. It is predicted that diabetes will affect 592 million people globally until 2035 (Daily et al., 2015). Diabetes is a non-transmissible chronic disease and a risk-factor to several other diseases; therefore, all efforts to control it should be employed since it could lead to positive impacts on the lives of millions of people and the public health system.

Ginger's anti-diabetic effects are related to insulin release and sensitivity to insulin, and carbohydrates metabolism. Its effects are also perceived on the late complications of diabetes involving liver, kidneys, eyes and the neural system (Li et al., 2012).

Shidfar et al., (2015) assessed the effects of ginger on type 2 diabetes patients supplemented with 3g of powder ginger for 3 months. Results revealed positive effects on daily glycemic indices and on the total antioxidant capacity. Since diabetes is related to oxidative stress, these are relevant results.

Venkateswaran et al., (2021) assessed anti-diabetic activity of polyphenolic extracts from Indian ginger cultivars and identified higher sensitivity to insulin and higher glucose intake in comparison with the control group.

Powdered ginger supplementation reduced serum glucose of type 2 diabetes patients, improving glucose homeostasis probably due to a reduction in insulin resistance (Choudhari e Kareppa, 2013).

How ginger improves glucose tolerance is not well understood. It is speculated that its pharmacological activity is related to its phenolic, polyphenolic and flavonoid components. There are indicatives that ginger reduces blood glucose through antagonistic activity against serotonin receptors and the inhibition of glucosidase and intestinal amylase (Gayar et al., 2019).

In summary, ginger is considered a safe and effective antidiabetic adjuvant with beneficial effects on lipid profile, insulin resistance and weight loss (Gayar et al., 2019).

Antioxidant Property

Oxidative stress is associated with non-transmissible chronic diseases (NTCD). The significant increase in morbimortality due to NTCD globally suggests that the strategies to promote health need innovations, especially when an ageing population is accompanied by an increase in NTCD (Seyedsadjadi Grant, 2021).

The antioxidant activity of spices such as ginger involves a series of phenomena that may include removal of free radicals, suppression of lipid peroxidation, stimulation of endogenous antioxidant enzymes, and inhibition of LDL oxidation and of the inducible nitric oxide synthase (Srinivasan, 2014).

Studies by Stoilova et al., (2007) indicate that the antioxidant activity of ginger rhizomes is higher than that of BHT (Butylated hydroxytoluene) and of the flavonoid quercetin, two highly effective antioxidants well-known by the pharmaceutical industry.

Anti-Inflammatory Property

The anti-inflammatory potential of ginger is related to its ability to inhibit metabolism or production of inflammatory markers. This biological activity may have several medicinal applications (Menon et al., 2021). Controlling inflammatory response is a key step in the treatment of non-transmissible chronic diseases (NTCD) (Chuengsamar et al., 2017).

Studies on animal models identified a probable mechanism of action involving the suppression of pro-inflammatory cytokines at the expression level (Kim et al., 2018).

Ginger also affects cyclooxygenase inhibitors, increasing its potential for the treatment of inflammatory diseases, such as rheumatoid arthritis (Funk et al., 2009).

Doses of ginger of 200mg/Kg significantly reduced incidence and severity of arthritis, production of pro-inflammatory cytokines and activated antioxidant defense (Ramadan, Kahtani and El-Sayed, 2011).

Raw extracts of ginger produced better results in inflammatory experimental models in comparison with isolated ginger bioactive compounds. The raw extract prevented late and early manifestations of standard inflammatory process for rheumatoid arthritis (Funk et al., 2009).

Protective Effects against Cancer

Many cancer therapies, such as chemotherapy, radiation and hormone treatments show several side effects. These effects jeopardize patient adhesion to treatment. It is important to identify natural compounds that are capable of not only enhancing standard treatment but also minimizing the effects of drugs (De Lima Silva et al., 2020).

Including phytochemicals in the patient's diet, especially in the early stages of the disease is a promising strategy. Among the phytochemicals studied with this aim, ginger receives a lot of attention due to its capacity to interfere with the onset and promotion of cancer (Hamza et al., 2021).

The protective effects against cancer are among its most studied properties. This effect is related to its anti-inflammatory, anti-tumor and antioxidant activities and involves tumor cell apoptosis and inhibition of cell proliferation (Miyosh et al., 2003).

In addition to its protective effects against cancer, ginger also helps to reduce the toxic effects of chemotherapy drugs (Menon, et al., 2021). 6-gingerol, one of ginger's bioactive compounds, showed cytotoxic activity against colon cancer cells (El-Naggar et al., 2017).

Ginger derivatives, either as isolates or extracts, showed anti-invasive, anti-proliferative, anti-metastatic and anti-tumor activities (De Lima et al., 2018).

In a study with rats, the group treated with ginger showed improvement in the general status, with dramatic decrease in number and incidence of dichromatic nodules, as well as in their growth rate. These effects were related to the apoptotic and anti-proliferative properties of ginger, that are specific for tumor cells (Hamza et al., 2021).

Final Considerations

Ginger has a great potential for health promotion, mainly due to its phenolic content since these compounds are related to control of non-transmissible chronic disease. The studies cited here point to the need to further investigate the use of ginger in health promotion.

References

Ali, B. H., Blunden, G., Tanira, M. O., Nemmar, A. Some phytochemical, pharmacological and toxicological properties of ginger (*Zingiber officinale* Roscoe): A review of recent research. *Food Chem Toxicol*, 46(2):409–420. 2008.

Choudhari, S. S., Kareppa, B. M. Identification of bioactive compounds of zingiber officinale roscoe rhizomes through gas chromatography and mass spectrometry. *Int J Pharm Res Dev*, 5, 16-20 .2013.

Christenhusz, M., Byng, J. W. The number of known plants species in the world and its annual increase. *Phytotaxa*, 261, 201–217. 2016.

Chuengsamar, N., S., Rattanamongkolgul, S., Sittithumcharee, G., Jirawatnotai, S. Association of serum high-sensitivity C-reactive protein with metabolic control and diabetic chronic vascular complications in patients with type 2 diabetes, *Diabetes & Metabol. Syndr.: Clini. Res. & Revi.* 11 (2) 103–108. 2017.

Daily, J. W., Yang, M., Kim, D. S., PARK, S. Efficacy of ginger for treating Type 2 diabetes: A systematic review and meta-analysis of randomized clinical trials. *Journal of Ethnic Foods*, 2 (1) 36-43. 2015.

De Lima, R. M. T., Dos Reis, A. C., De Menezes, A. P. M., Santos, J. V. O., Filho, J., Ferreira, J. R. O., De Alencar, M., Da Mata, A., Khan, I. N., Islam, A., Uddin, S. J., Ali, E. S., Islam, M. T., Tripathi, S., Mishra, S. K., Mubarak, M. S., Melo- Cavalcante, A. A. C. Protective and therapeutic potential of ginger (*Zingiber officinale*) extract and [6]-gingerol in cancer: A comprehensive review. *Phytotherapy Research*, 32(10), 1885–1907. 2018.

De Lima Silva, W. C., Conti, R., De Almeida, L. C., Morais, P. A. B., Borges, K. B., Júnior, V. L., Costa-Lotufo, L. V., De Souza Borges, W. Novel [6]-gingerol Triazole Derivatives and their Antiproliferative Potential against Tumor Cells. *Curr Top Med Chem*, 20(2):161-169. 2020.

El-Naggar, M. H., Mira, A., Bar, F. M. A., Shimizu, K., Amer, M. M., Badria, F. A. Synthesis, docking, cytotoxicity, and LTA4H inhibitory activity of new gingerol derivatives as potential colorectal cancer therapy, *Bioorganic & Medicinal Chemistry*, 25, 3: 1277-1285 . 2017.

Funk, J. L., Frye, J. B., Oyarzo, J. N. Timmermann, B. N. Comparative effects of two gingerol-containing *Zingiber officinale* extracts on experimental rheumatoid Arthritis, *J. Nat. Prod.* 72, 403–407. 2009.

Gayar, M. H. E., Aboromia, M. M. M., Ibrahim, N. A., Hafiz, M. Hu. A. Effects of ginger powder supplementation on glycemic status and lipid profile in newly diagnosed obese patients with type 2 diabetes mellitus. *Obesity Medicine*, 14. 2019.

Getaneh, A., Guadie, A., Tefera, M. Levels of heavy metals in ginger (*Zingiber officinale* Roscoe*) from selected districts of Central Gondar Zone, Ethiopia and associated health risk. *Heliyon*, 7, 4. 2021

Ghafoor, A., Juhaimi, F. A., Özcan, M. M., Uslu, N., Babiker, E. E., Ahmed, I. A. M. Total phenolics, total carotenoids, individual phenolics and antioxidant activity of ginger (*Zingiber officinale*) rhizome as affected by drying methods. *LWT*, 126. 2020.

Hamza, A. A., Heeba, G. H., Hamza, S., Abdalla, A., Amin A. Standardized extract of ginger ameliorates liver cancer by reducing proliferation and inducing apoptosis through inhibition oxidative stress/ inflammation pathway *Biomedicine & Pharmacotherapy*, 134: 111-102. 2021.

Idris, N. A., Yasin, H. M., Usmana. Voltammetric and spectroscopic determination of polyphenols and antioxidants in ginger (*Zingiber officinale* Roscoe), *Heliyon*, 5: 5. 2019.

Jafarnejad, S., Keshavarz, S. A., Mahbubi, S., Saremi, S., Arab, A., Abbasi, S., Djafarian, K. Effect of ginger (*Zingiber officinale*) on blood glucose and lipid concentrations in diabetic and hyperlipidemic subjects: A meta-analysis of randomized controlled trials. *Journal of Functional Foods*, 29:127-134. 2017.

Kim, S., Lee, M. S., Jung, S., Son, H. Y., Park, S., Kang, B., Kim, S. Y., Kim, I.-H., Kim, C. T., Kim, Y. Ginger extract ameliorates obesity and inflammation via regulating MicroRNA-21/132 expression and AMPK activation in white adipose tissue. *Nutrients*, 10 (11): 1567. 2018.

Li, H., Liu, Y., Luo, D., Ma, Y., Zhang, J., Li, M., Yao, L., Shi, X., Liu, X., Yang, K. Ginger for health care: An overview of systematic reviews. *Complement Ther Med.* Aug;45:114-123. 2019.

Li, Y., Tran, V. H., Duke, C. C., Roufogalis, B. D. Preventive and protective properties of *Zingiber officinale* (Ginger) in *diabetes mellitus*, diabetic complications, and associated lipid and other metabolic disorders: a brief review, *Evid. Based Complement. Alternat. Med.* 2012.

Mao, Q. Q., Xu, X. Y., Cao, S. Y., Gan, R. Y., Corke, H., Beta, T., Li, H. B. Bioactive compounds and bioactivities of ginger (*Zingiber officinale* Roscoe). *Foods*, 8 (6), 185. 2019.

Menon, V., Elgharib, M., El-Awad, R., Saleh, E. Ginger: From serving table to salient therapy. Food *Bioscience*, 41, 2021.

Miyoshi, N., Nakamura, Y., Ueda, Y., Abe, M., Ozawa, Y., Uchida, K., Osawa, T. Dietary ginger constituents, galanals A and B, are potent apoptosis inducers in Human T lymphoma Jurkat cells. *Cancer Lett.* Sep 25;199(2):113-119. 2003.

Prakash, U. N., Srinivasan, K. Fat digestion and absorption in spice-pretreated rats. *J Sci Food Agric.* Feb;92(3):503-510.2012.

Ramadan, G., Al-Kahtani, M. A., El-Sayed, W. M. Anti-inflammatory and anti-oxidant properties of Curcuma longa (turmeric) versus *Zingiber officinale* (ginger) rhizomes in rat adjuvant-induced arthritis. *Inflammation*. Aug;34(4):291-301.2011.

Ravindran, P. N., & Babu, K.). *Ginger: The genus zingiber*. Florida: CRC Press, 2016. ISBN 9780415324687.

Sang, S., Snook, H. D., Tareq, F. S., Fasina, Y. Precision research on ginger: The type of ginger matters. *Journal of Agricultural and Food Chemistry*, 68(32), 8517–8523. 2020.

Shidfar, F., Rajab, A., Rahideh, T., Khandouzi, N., Hosseini, S., Shidfar, S. The effect of ginger (*Zingiber officinale*) on glycemic markers in patients with type 2 diabetes. *J Complement Integr Med.* Jun;12(2):165-170. 2015.

SI, W., Chen, Y. P., Zhang, J., Chen, Z. Y., Chung, H. Y. Antioxidant activities of ginger extract and its constituents toward lipids. *Food Chem.* Jan 15;239:1117-1125. 2018.

Srinivasan, K. Antioxidant potential of spices and their active constituents, *Crit. Rev. Food Sci. Nutr.* 54, 352–372. 2014.

Srinivasan, K. Ginger rhizomes (*Zingiber officinale*): A spice with multiple health beneficial potentials. *PharmaNutrition*. 5(1):18–28. 2017.

Seyedsadjadi, N.; Grant, R. The Potential Benefit of Monitoring Oxidative Stress and Inflammation in the Prevention of Non-Communicable Diseases (NCDs). *Antioxidants*, 10, 15. 2021.

Stoilova, I., Krastanov, A., Stoyanova, A., Denev, P., Gargova, S. Antioxidant activity of a ginger extract (*Zingiber officinale*). *Food Chem*, 102, 764– 770. 2007.

Teng, H., Seuseu, K. T., Lee, W-Y., Chen, L. Comparing the effects of microwave radiation on 6-gingerol and 6-shogaol from ginger rhizomes (*Zingiber officinale* Rosc). *PLoS ONE* 14(6). 2019.

Ujang, Z., Nordin, N., Subramaniam, T. Ginger species and their traditional uses in modern applications. *Journal of Industrial Technology*, 23, 59–70. 2015.

United States Department of Agriculture. *Natural Resources Conservation Service: Classification.* Disponível em: http://plants. usda.gov/core/profile?symbol=ZIOF. Acesso em: 21/06/2021.

Venkateswaran, M., Jayabal, S., Hemaiswarya, S., Murugesan, S., Enkateswara, S., Doble, M., Periyasamy, S. Polyphenol-rich Indian ginger cultivars ameliorate GLUT4 activity in C2C12 cells, inhibit diabetes-related enzymes and LPS-induced inflammation: An in vitro study. *Journal of Food Biochemistry*, Article e13600. 2021.

Bibliography

101 amazing uses for garlic: prevent colds, ease seasickness, repair glass, and 98 more!

LCCN	2018936022
Type of material	Book
Personal name	Branson, Susan, author.
Main title	101 amazing uses for garlic: prevent colds, ease seasickness, repair glass, and 98 more! / Susan Branson.
Edition	First edition.
Published/Produced	[Sanger, CA]: Familius LLC, 2018. ©2018
Description	141 pages; 21 cm.
ISBN	9781945547911 paperback
	194554791X paperback
LC classification	RM666.G15 B73 2018
Variant title	One hundred and one amazing uses for garlic
	Hundred and one amazing uses for garlic
Summary	COMPLEMENTARY THERAPIES, HEALING & HEALTH. It turns out that garlic does more than keep away vampires! Garlic is a natural anti-inflammatory, antibiotic, antifungal, and antiparasitic agent. With benefits ranging from slowing collagen depletion and battling cancer cells to preventing hair loss and providing relief for a cold, garlic is a must-have for your kitchen and your everyday life. Millions of people are turning away from the harsh effects of modern solutions and back to the gentle but powerful benefits of nature's oldest remedies. In her 101 Amazing Uses series, Susan

	Branson, a holistic nutritional consultant, expertly outlines 101 incredible uses for everyday ingredients like garlic, apple cider vinegar, ginger, and coconut oil.-- Source other than the Library of Congress.
Subjects	Garlic--Therapeutic use.
	Spices--Therapeutic use.
	Cooking (Garlic)
	Cooking (Garlic)
	Garlic--Therapeutic use.
	Spices--Therapeutic use.
Notes	Includes bibliographical references.

101 Amazing uses for honey: clean scrapes & cuts, soften your skin, make a soothing bath, and 98 more!

LCCN	2018937189
Type of material	Book
Personal name	Branson, Susan (Holistic nutritional consultant), author.
Main title	101 Amazing uses for honey: clean scrapes & cuts, soften your skin, make a soothing bath, and 98 more! / Susan Branson.
Edition	First edition.
Published/Produced	[United States]: Familius LLC, [2019]
	©2019
Description	150 pages; 21 cm.
ISBN	9781641700443 (paperback)
	1641700440 (paperback)
LC classification	RM666.H55 B73 2019
Variant title	Hundred and one uses for honey
	One hundred and one uses for honey
Summary	"Honey: this sweet, golden nectar with a low glycemic index has made a big comeback as a natural sweetener. But honey isn't just to sweeten your tea! Its incredible health benefits range from treating anemia to increasing calcium absorption to fighting off colds! Holistic nutritional consultant Susan Branson provides 101 useful and scientifically documented reasons to add honey to

your diet and daily life. Millions of people are turning away from the harsh effects of modern solutions and back to the gentle but powerful benefits of nature's oldest remedies. In her 101 Amazing Uses series, Susan Branson, a holistic nutritional consultant, expertly outlines 101 incredible uses for apple cider vinegar, ginger, essential oils, coconut oil, and more. Each book is divided into tabbed sections filled with a total of 101 easy-to-read, bite-sized benefits for everything from health to beauty to household cleaning. Promote healthy skin, reduce stress, boost your metabolism, tenderize meat, and more with these simple, accessible, natural solutions."-- Cataloguer.

Subjects	Honey--Therapeutic use.
	Natural foods--Health aspects.
	Honey--Health aspects.
	Honey--Therapeutic use.
	Natural foods--Health aspects.
Notes	Includes bibliographical references.
Series	A 101 amazing uses book
	Branson, Suan (Holistic nutritional consultant) 101 amazing uses book.

101 amazing uses for turmeric: reduce joint pain, soothe your stomach, make a delicious dinner, and 98 more!

LCCN	2018936021
Type of material	Book
Personal name	Branson, Susan, author.
Main title	101 amazing uses for turmeric: reduce joint pain, soothe your stomach, make a delicious dinner, and 98 more! / Susan Branson.
Edition	First edition.
Published/Produced	[United States]: Familius, [2018]
Description	143 pages; 21 cm
ISBN	1945547928 (paperback)
LC classification	RS165.T8 B737 2018
Variant title	One hundred and one amazing uses for turmeric
	One hundred one amazing uses for turmeric

Summary	Turmeric gives traditional curry its vibrant flavor and yellow color, but did you know this spice has been used medicinally in India for centuries? Research suggests turmeric can improve brain function, tame heartburn, prevent inflammation, and provide many other health benefits. Millions of people are turning away from the harsh effects of modern solutions and back to the gentle but powerful benefits of nature's oldest remedies. In her 101 Amazing Uses series, Susan Branson, a holistic nutritional consultant, expertly outlines 101 incredible uses for everyday ingredients like garlic, apple cider vinegar, ginger, and coconut oil. Each book is divided into tabbed sections filled with a total of 101 easy-to-read, bite-size benefits for everything from health to beauty to household cleaning. Promote healthy skin, reduce stress, boost your metabolism, tenderize meat, and more with these simple, accessible, natural solutions!-- Source other than Library of Congress.
Contents	Alleviate illness and infection -- Attain physical and mental wellness -- Accentuate beauty -- Apply in arts and crafts.
Subjects	Turmeric--Therapeutic use. Turmeric.
Notes	Includes bibliographical references.

Alchemy of herbs: transform everyday ingredients into foods & remedies that heal

LCCN	2016037604
Type of material	Book
Personal name	Forêt, Rosalee de la, 1980- author.
Main title	Alchemy of herbs: transform everyday ingredients into foods & remedies that heal / Rosalee de la Forêt.
Published/Produced	Carlsbad, California: Hay House, Inc., [2017] ©2017
Description	xxi, 355 pages: color illustrations; 24 cm
ISBN	9781401950064 (paperback) 140195006X (paperback)

LC classification	RM666.H33 F664 2017
Summary	"Just as alchemists transform the ordinary into the extraordinary, with this book you can transform everyday herbs and spices into effective healing herbal remedies. Rosalee de la Foret, a clinical herbalist and education director at LearningHerbs.com, examines the history and modern-day use of 29 herbs, offering clinical studies to support their healing properties. She also dives into the energetics of herbalism, teaching readers how to match the properties of each plant to their unique needs, for a truly personalized approach to health. The recipes in this book take a variety of forms--from teas, salves, and pastilles to beauty products and delicious foods--to show how easy it is to incorporate the healing power of herbs into your everyday life. You could start your day with Spiced Cold Brew Coffee, pamper your skin with Green Tea and Rose Facial Cream, make a meal of Astragalus Bone Broth and Sage Chicken, then treat yourself to Cardamom Chocolate Mousse Cake and a Holy Basil-Ginger Julep. Beautiful photos taken by the author of the herbs and recipes complement each chapter. This book will appeal to those interested in natural health and herbalism, and the recipes offer an easy entry for beginners. Readers will never look at cinnamon, coffee, parsley, lavender, or even chocolate the same way as they realize the kitchen can be their medicine cabinet"-- Provided by publisher.
Contents	Your introduction to herbs and spices. The benefits of herbs and spices -- How do we know herbs can do that? -- Matching herbs to you- not to an ailment -- How to get the most out of this book -- The herbs. Pungent. Black pepper -- Cayenne -- Cinnamon -- Fennel -- Garlic -- Ginger -- Holy basil -- Lavender -- Mustard -- Nutmeg -- Parsley -- Peppermint -- Rosemary -- Sage -- Thyme -- Turmeric -- Salty. Nettle -- Sour. Elder -- Hawthorn -- Lemon balm --

	Rose -- Tea -- Bitter. Artichoke -- Cacao -- Chamomile -- Coffee -- Dandelion -- Sweet. Ashwagandha -- Astragalus.
Subjects	Herbs--Therapeutic use--Popular works.
	Self-care, Health--Popular works.
	Holistic medicine--Popular works.
	Health & Fitness / Herbal Medications.
	Medical / Holistic Medicine.
	Cooking / Specific Ingredients / Herbs, Spices, Condiments.
Notes	Includes bibliographical references (pages 325-327) and index.

Anti-inflammatory drinks for health: 100 smoothies, shots, teas, broths, and seltzers to help prevent disease, lose weight, increase energy, look radiant, reduce pain, and more!

LCCN	2018055602
Type of material	Book
Personal name	Flaherty, Maryea, author.
Main title	Anti-inflammatory drinks for health: 100 smoothies, shots, teas, broths, and seltzers to help prevent disease, lose weight, increase energy, look radiant, reduce pain, and more! / Maryea Flaherty.
Edition	First Adams Media trade paperback edition.
Published/Produced	New York: Adams Media, 2019.
Description	159 pages: color illustrations; 24 cm.
ISBN	9781507209585 (paperback)
	1507209584 (paperback)
	(ebook)
	(ebook)
LC classification	RB131 .F53 2019
Summary	"100 delicious drink recipes packed with nutrients scientifically proven to reduce inflammation--perfect for both enthusiasts of natural health and those new to its benefits. Chronic inflammation is a major health risk. Studies have shown it wreaks havoc on your body and contributes to heart disease, diabetes, Alzheimer's--and even cancer. And diet--specifically one high in processed, fatty, and sugary

foods--is one of the main causes of chronic inflammation. But preventing and/or reducing inflammation can be easy as making a delicious drink--let this book show you how! Anti-Inflammatory Drinks for Health contains 100 great-tasting recipes for drinks packed with anti-inflammatory foods including cinnamon, tart cherries, ginger, turmeric, blueberries, and many more. In addition to helping reduce the risk of developing disease, these drinks also can aid in: -Weight loss -Increasing energy -Reducing pain -Slowing the signs of aging Also included is a list of inflammatory foods to avoid and even more ideas for how to add inflammation-fighting foods to any diet! Improve your diet, your health, and your life, with Anti-Inflammatory Drinks for Health!"-- Provided by publisher.

"Chronic inflammation is a major health risk. Studies have shown it wreaks havoc on your body and contributes to heart disease, diabetes, Alzheimer's--and even cancer. But preventing and/or reducing inflammation can be easy as making a delicious drink--let this book show you how! Anti-Inflammatory Drinks for Health contains 100 great-tasting recipes for drinks packed with anti-inflammatory foods including cinnamon, tart cherries, ginger, turmeric, blueberries, and many more. In addition to helping reduce the risk of developing disease, these drinks also can aid in: weight loss; increasing energy; reducing pain; and more"-- Provided by publisher.

Subjects   Inflammation--Diet therapy.
Inflammation--Diet therapy--Recipes.
Cooking / Health & Healing / General.
Cooking / Beverages / Non-Alcoholic.
Health & Fitness / Alternative Therapies.

Notes   "Enjoy great benefits and great taste!"
Includes index.

Series   For health

Behavioral healthcare and technology: using science-based innovations to transform practice

LCCN	2014028147
Type of material	Book
Main title	Behavioral healthcare and technology: using science-based innovations to transform practice / edited by Lisa A. Marsch, PhD, Sarah E. Lord, PhD, Jesse Dallery, PhD.
Published/Produced	Oxford; New York: Oxford University Press, 2015.
Description	xvi, 348 pages: illustrations; 27 cm
ISBN	9780199314027 (hbk.: acid-free paper)
	0199314020 (hbk.: acid-free paper)
LC classification	R855.3 .B45 2015
Related names	Marsch, Lisa A., editor.
	Lord, Sarah E. (Sarah Elizabeth), editor.
	Dallery, Jesse, editor.
Contents	Technology and the stage model of behavioral intervention development / Lisa S. Onken, Varda Shoham -- Theoretical models to inform technology-based health behavior interventions / William T. Riley -- Behavioral monitoring and assessment via sensing technologies / Santosh Kumar, J. Gayle Beck, Emre Ertin, Marcia Scott -- Technology-based behavioral interventions for alcohol and drug use problems / Aimee Campbell, Frederick Muench, Edward V. Nunes -- Using behavioral intervention technologies to reduce the burden of mood and anxiety disorders / Stephen M. Schueller, Miraj Chokshi, David C. Mohr -- Technologies for people with serious mental illness / Dror Ben-Zeev, Robert E. Drake, Rachel M. Brian -- Applying technology to medication management and adherence / Leah L. Zullig, Ryan J. Shaw, Hayden B. Bosworth -- Technological approaches to assess and treat cigarette smoking / Jesse Dallery, Sarah Martner -- Technology-based interventions to promote diet, exercise and weight control / Deborah Tate, Carmina Valle -- Evidence-based approaches to harnessing technology to provide social-

emotional support / Timothy Bickmore -- mHealth analytics / Daniel M. Smith, Theodore A. Walls -- Research designs to develop and evaluate technology-based health behavior interventions / Jesse Dallery, William Riley, Inbal Nahum-Shani -- Evaluating mechanisms of behavior change to inform and evaluate technology-based interventions / Amanda N. Baraldi, Ingrid C. Wurpts, David P. MacKinnon, Ginger Lockhart -- Economics analysis of technology-based behavioral health care systems / Daniel Polsky -- Models for effective dissemination and implementation of technology-based behavioral health care systems / Sarah Lord -- Privacy, security, and regulatory considerations as related to behavioral health information technology / Penelope P. Hughes, Melissa M. Goldstein -- Harnessing mHealth in low-resource settings to overcome health system constraints and achieve universal access to health / Garrett Mehl, Lavanya Vasudevan, Lianne Gonsalves, Matt Berg, Tamsyn Seimon, Marleen Temmerman, Alain Labrique -- Open architecture and standards in mobile health / Julia E. Hoffman, Kelly M. Ramsey, Deborah Estrin -- Using technology to integrate behavioral health into primary care / Lola Awoyinka, David H. Gustafson, Roberta Johnson -- The potential of technology solutions for behavioral healthcare disparities / Michael Christopher Gibbons -- Behavioral health information technology adoption in the context of a changing healthcare landscape / Wendy Nilsen, Misha Pavel -- Envisioning the future: transformation of health care systems via technology / Lisa A. Marsch.

Subjects Biomedical Technology.
Mental Disorders--therapy.
Mental Health Services--organization & administration.

Notes Includes bibliographical references and index.

Bioactive compounds of medicinal plants: properties and potential for human health

LCCN	2018024978
Type of material	Book
Main title	Bioactive compounds of medicinal plants: properties and potential for human health / editors, Megh R. Goyal, Ademola Olabode Ayeleso.
Published/Produced	Toronto; New Jersey: Apple Academic Press, 2018.
Description	1 online resource.
ISBN	9781315147475 ()
LC classification	RS164
Related names	Goyal, Megh R., editor.
	Ayeleso, Ademola Olabode, editor.
Contents	Phytochemistry and antifungal activity of desmodium adscendens root extracts / Nwanekwu Kenneth Emeka, Adeniyi Bola, and Mahady Gail -- Bioactive compounds in plants and their antioxidant capacity / Oluyemisi E. Adelakun, Islamiyat Folashade Bolarinwa, and Johnson Akinwumi Adejuyitan -- Plants of the genus Syzygium (Myrtaceae): a review on ethnobotany, medicinal properties, and phytochemistry / Ian Edwin Cock and Matthew Cheesman -- Effects of Talinum triangulare on hepatic antioxidant gene expression profile in carbon tetrachloride-induced rat liver injury / Gbenga Anthony Adefolaju, Benedict Abiola Falana, Adeoye Oluwole Oyewopo, and Anthony Mwakikunga -- Review on potential of seeds and value-added products of Bambara groundnut (Vigna subterranea): antioxidant, anti-inflammatory, and anti-oxidative stress / Yvonne Yeukai Murevanhema, Victoria Adaora Jideani, and Oluwafemi Omoniyi Oguntibeju -- Antioxidant and antimicrobial activity of Opuntia aurantiaca Lindl / Wilfred Mbeng Otang and Anthony Jide Afolayan -- Dietary Intervention of Utazi (Gongrenema latifolium) supplemented diet using wistar male rat animal brain model / Esther Emem Nwanna, Ganiyu Oboh, and Olukemi Abimbola Okediran --

	Therapeutic potentials of selected medicinal plants in the management of diabetes mellitus: a review / Folorunso Adewale Olabiyi, Yapo Guillaume Aboua, and Oluwafemi Omoniyi Oguntibeju -- Medicinal activities of Anchomanes difformis and its potential in the treatment of diabetes mellitus and other disease conditions: a review / Toyin D. Udje, Nicole L. Brooks, and Oluwafemi O. Oguntibeju -- Screening of different extracts of Ageratum conyzoides for inhibition of diabetes-related enzymes / Mutiu I. Kazeem, Oluwatosin O. Ogunkelu, Ademola O. Ayeleso, and Emmanuel Mukwevho -- Potential of Catharanthus roseus and Punica granatum in the management and treatment of diabetes mellitus and its complications / Mediline Goboza, Prisca Kachepe, Yapo Guillaume Aboua, and Oluwafemi Omoniyi Oguntibeju -- Ginger and turmeric supplemented diet as a novel dietary approach for management of hypertension: a review / Ayodele Jacob Akinyemi, Ganiyu Oboh, and Maria Rosa Chitolina Schetinger.
Subjects	Plants, Medicinal Phytotherapy Diabetes Mellitus--drug therapy Plant Extracts--therapeutic use Africa
Notes	Includes bibliographical references and index. Description based on print version record and CIP data provided by publisher; resource not viewed.
Additional formats	Print version: Bioactive compounds of medicinal plants Toronto; New Jersey: Apple Academic Press, 2018 9781771886482 (DLC) 2018024233
Series	Innovations in plant science for better health: from soil to fork

Bioactive compounds of medicinal plants: properties and potential for human health

LCCN	2018024233
Type of material	Book

Bibliography

Main title	Bioactive compounds of medicinal plants: properties and potential for human health / editors, Megh R. Goyal, Ademola Olabode Ayeleso.
Published/Produced	Toronto; New Jersey: Apple Academic Press, 2018.
ISBN	9781771886482 (hardcover: alk. paper)
LC classification	RS164
Related names	Goyal, Megh R., editor.
	Ayeleso, Ademola Olabode, editor.
Contents	Phytochemistry and antifungal activity of desmodium adscendens root extracts / Nwanekwu Kenneth Emeka, Adeniyi Bola, and Mahady Gail -- Bioactive compounds in plants and their antioxidant capacity / Oluyemisi E. Adelakun, Islamiyat Folashade Bolarinwa, and Johnson Akinwumi Adejuyitan -- Plants of the genus Syzygium (Myrtaceae): a review on ethnobotany, medicinal properties, and phytochemistry / Ian Edwin Cock and Matthew Cheesman -- Effects of Talinum triangulare on hepatic antioxidant gene expression profile in carbon tetrachloride-induced rat liver injury / Gbenga Anthony Adefolaju, Benedict Abiola Falana, Adeoye Oluwole Oyewopo, and Anthony Mwakikunga -- Review on potential of seeds and value-added products of Bambara groundnut (Vigna subterranea): antioxidant, anti-inflammatory, and anti-oxidative stress / Yvonne Yeukai Murevanhema, Victoria Adaora Jideani, and Oluwafemi Omoniyi Oguntibeju -- Antioxidant and antimicrobial activity of Opuntia aurantiaca Lindl / Wilfred Mbeng Otang and Anthony Jide Afolayan -- Dietary Intervention of Utazi (Gongrenema latifolium) supplemented diet using wistar male rat animal brain model / Esther Emem Nwanna, Ganiyu Oboh, and Olukemi Abimbola Okediran -- Therapeutic potentials of selected medicinal plants in the management of diabetes mellitus: a review / Folorunso Adewale Olabiyi, Yapo Guillaume Aboua, and Oluwafemi Omoniyi Oguntibeju -- Medicinal activities of Anchomanes difformis and

	its potential in the treatment of diabetes mellitus and other disease conditions: a review / Toyin D. Udje, Nicole L. Brooks, and Oluwafemi O. Oguntibeju -- Screening of different extracts of Ageratum conyzoides for inhibition of diabetes-related enzymes / Mutiu I. Kazeem, Oluwatosin O. Ogunkelu, Ademola O. Ayeleso, and Emmanuel Mukwevho -- Potential of Catharanthus roseus and Punica granatum in the management and treatment of diabetes mellitus and its complications / Mediline Goboza, Prisca Kachepe, Yapo Guillaume Aboua, and Oluwafemi Omoniyi Oguntibeju -- Ginger and turmeric supplemented diet as a novel dietary approach for management of hypertension: a review / Ayodele Jacob Akinyemi, Ganiyu Oboh, and Maria Rosa Chitolina Schetinger.
Subjects	Plants, Medicinal Phytotherapy Diabetes Mellitus--drug therapy Plant Extracts--therapeutic use Africa
Notes	Includes bibliographical references and index.
Additional formats	Online version: Bioactive compounds of medicinal plants Toronto; New Jersey: Apple Academic Press, 2018 9781315147475 (DLC) 2018024978
Series	Innovations in plant science for better health: from soil to fork Innovations in plant science for better health.

Biology and pathogenesis of rhabdo- and filoviruses

LCCN	2014042992
Type of material	Book
Main title	Biology and pathogenesis of rhabdo- and filoviruses / editors, Asit K. Pattnaik, University of Nebraska-Lincoln, USA, Michael A. Whitt, University of Tennessee Health Science Center, USA.
Published/Produced	New Jersey: World Scientific, [2015]
Description	x, 627 pages: illustrations (some color), color maps; 24 cm

ISBN	9789814635332 (hardback: alk. paper)
	9814635332 (hardback: alk. paper)
LC classification	QR415 .B56 2015
Related names	Pattnaik, Asit Kumar, editor.
	Whitt, Michael A., editor.
Contents	Overview of rhabdo- and filoviruses / Asit K. Pattnaik and Michael A. Whitt -- Rhabdovirus structure / Ming Luo -- The pathway of VSV entry into cells / Shem Johnson and Jean Gruenberg -- Rhabdovirus glycoproteins / Yves Gaudin and Michael A. Whitt -- VSV RNA transcription and replication / Jacques Perrault -- Host cell functions in vesicular stomatitis virus replication / Phat X. Dinh, Anshuman Das, and Asit K. Pattnaik -- Cytopathogenesis of rhabdoviruses / Douglas S. Lyles -- Assembly and budding of rhabdo- and filoviruses / Ziying Han and Ronald N. Harty -- Rhabdoviruses as vaccine vectors from initial development to clinical trials / John K. Rose and David K. Clarke -- Oncolytic rhabdoviruses / Nicole E. Forbes and John C. Bell -- Use of rhabdoviruses to study neural circuitry / Melanie Ginger, Guillaume Bony, Matthias Haber, and Andreas Frick -- Evolution of rhabdo- and filoviruses / Isabel S. Novella, John B. Presloid, and R. Travis Taylor -- Emerging rhabdoviruses / Imke Steffen and Graham Simmons -- Rabies virus replication and pathogenesis / Andrew W. Hudacek and Matthias J. Schnell -- Activation and evasion of innate immune response by rhabdoviruses / Karl-Klaus Conzelmann -- Rabies virus vaccines / Ying Huang, Clement W. Gnanadurai, and Zhen F. Fu -- Filovirus structure and morphogenesis / Timothy F. Booth, Daniel Beniac, Melissa Rabb, and Lindsey Lamboo -- Epidemiology and pathogenesis of filovirus infections / Logan Banadyga and Hideki Ebihara -- Filovirus entry into susceptible cells / Rohit K. Jangra, Eva Mittler, and Kartik Chandran -- Filovirus transcription & replication / Kristina

	Brauburger, Laure R. Deflubé, and Elke Muhlberger -- Innate immune evasion mechanisms of filoviruses / Christopher F. Basler, Gaya K. Amarasinghe, and Daisy W. Leung -- Vaccines and antivirals for filoviruses / Chad E. Mire & Thomas W. Geisbert.
Subjects	Rhabdoviridae--physiology.
	Filoviridae--pathogenicity.
	Filoviridae--physiology.
	Rhabdoviridae--pathogenicity.
Notes	Includes bibliographical references and index.

Clean green eats: 100+ clean-eating recipes to improve your whole life

LCCN	2015009848
Type of material	Book
Personal name	Kumai, Candice.
Main title	Clean green eats: 100+ clean-eating recipes to improve your whole life / Candice Kumai.
Edition	First edition.
Published/Produced	Broadway, New York: HarperWave, [2015]
Description	xiii, 287 pages: illustrations; 23 cm
ISBN	9780062388735 (hardback)
LC classification	TX801 .K86 2015
Summary	"Clean up your diet and look and feel better than ever with this simple, beautiful cookbook featuring more than 100 recipes that make it easy and delicious to eat clean and green. We all know we should eat more green foods, but after a few variations on the same salad, juice or smoothie, it's easy to run out of ideas that excite our taste buds. In Clean Green Eats, celebrity chef Candice Kumai offers an answer to that dilemma, offering more than 100 simple, unique and delicious recipes made from whole foods packed with of nutrients that will help you lose weight, detox, and look amazing. All of her recipes are effortlessly gluten free (no complicated ingredients required!) and while a plant-based diet is the focus, the idea of "meat as a treat"--eating high-quality, sensible portions of animal protein--is also central to her plan. Clean Green Eats kicks off with

	Candice's one week cleanse, which includes juices, smoothies, and simple meals, and continues with a six-week plan to develop healthy practices that will last a lifetime. There's no deprivation with Candice's delicious drinks, breakfasts, snacks, soups, salads, sides, mains, and desserts. Start your day with a Coconut Almond Green Smooth or Cinnamon-Spiced Granola. For lunch, fill up on Farro, Edamame, and Pea Salad. Whip up Asian Ginger Garlic Steak Salad, Superfood Curry Salmon Salad, or Chili Lime Shrimp Tostadas for a delicious dinner. For a fabulous finale, she includes desserts like Vegan Dark-Chocolate Avocado Cake and Banana Chocolate Chip Cookie Dough 'Ice Cream.'Banish the processed food, sugar, and carb habits that lead to fatigue, belly bloat, poor digestion, and constant cravings--let Clean Green Eats help you look and feel better than ever, no deprivation required!"-- Provided by publisher.
	"A simple and beautiful guide to cleaning up your diet and eating more greens with more than 100 delicious recipes to help you lose weight, get great skin, and stay healthy"-- Provided by publisher.
Subjects	Cooking (Vegetables)
	Vegetable juices.
	Nutrition.
	Detoxification (Health)
	Self-care, Health.

Clean-eating breakfasts and lunches made simple: 75 flavorful and nutritious recipes that ditch processed ingredients

LCCN	2019932080
Type of material	Book
Personal name	Baier, Lacey, author.
Main title	Clean-eating breakfasts and lunches made simple: 75 flavorful and nutritious recipes that ditch processed ingredients / Lacey Baier.
Published/Produced	Salem, MA: Page Street Publishing Co., 2019. ©2019

Description	192 pages: color illustrations; 23 cm
ISBN	9781624148408 (softcover)
	1624148409 (softcover)
LC classification	TX741 .B325 2019
Summary	Stick to Your Health Goals with Easy, Wholesome Meals. Lacey Baier, founder of the clean-eating blog A Sweet Pea Chef, brings you a wide variety of fun, satisfying breakfasts and lunches to help you eat clean--and stay healthy--all day long. By ditching refined sugars and harmful additives and adding in natural sweeteners and low-carb, high-protein foods, you never have to give up the meals you love to eat. Every one of these fuss-free, nutrient-packed dishes comes together quickly, and most can be prepped the night before. Never skip breakfast again with filling grab-and-go options like Bananas Foster Overnight Oats or the Blackberry Cobbler Greek Yogurt Bowl. Say goodbye to expensive, unhealthy deli sandwiches and reach for preservative-free lunches that are anything but boring like the Chickpea Meatballs Sub and Rainbow Detox Salad with Sesame-Ginger Peanut Dressing. Lacey shares smart tips and provides support for making healthy choices, because she's been there! Her delicious recipes make the clean-eating lifestyle easy, convenient and enjoyable.
Contents	Satisfying breakfast bowls -- On the griddle: low-carb, high-protein pancakes and waffles -- Beyond basic oatmeal: delicious prep-ahead overnight oats -- Easy power-packed smoothies -- Grab-'n'-go muffins and breakfast bars -- Fun breakfasts for your inner child -- Classic comfort food made clean -- Exciting and vibrant salads -- Lunch bowls of goodness -- Shockingly healthy appetizers you can enjoy as a lunch -- Delicious, nutritious, piled-high sandwiches.
Subjects	Cooking (Natural foods)
	Breakfasts.
	Luncheons.

	Cooking / General.
	Breakfasts.
	Cooking (Natural foods)
	Luncheons.
Form/Genre	Cookbooks.
	Cookbooks.
Notes	Includes index.

Coconut. ginger. shrimp. rum.: Caribbean flavors for every season

LCCN	2016043430
Type of material	Book
Personal name	Washington, Brigid, author.
Main title	Coconut. ginger. shrimp. rum.: Caribbean flavors for every season / Brigid Washington.
Published/Produced	New York: Skyhorse Publishing, 2017.
Description	xv, 126 pages: color illustrations; 25 cm
ISBN	9781510714939 (hardback)
LC classification	TX716.A1 W37 2017
Summary	"The recipes in this book will highlight seasonal bounties and four major Caribbean flavors, resulting in a basketful of healthy recipes (many vegetarian), which the author refers to as "edible treasures." This innovative cookbook presents a new way to look at the four seasons through four ingredients that are integral to Caribbean flavors and culture, but available everywhere. Coconut, ginger, shrimp, and rum each boast unique health benefits, but are still simple and fundamental ingredients that will take any cook through the year, and especially highlighting seasonal ingredients! The book is divided into four seasons, and each of those is divided into "Light Fare," "Mains," "To Sip," and "Sweets." Recipes include: Coconut spiced cashews White coconut gazpacho Rum buttered jerk wings Spring pea and ginger risotto Rhubarb & ginger challah Salsa verde coconut rice Grilled strawberry ginger shortcake Garlicky parmesan shrimp & fava bean ravioli Poached pear negroni"-- Provided by publisher.

Subjects	Cooking, Caribbean. Cooking, West Indian. Seasonal cooking--Caribbean Area. Cooking / Regional & Ethnic / Caribbean & West Indian.
Form/Genre	Cookbooks.

Ethnopharmacological investigation of Indian spices

LCCN	2019040959
Type of material	Book
Main title	Ethnopharmacological investigation of Indian spices / Neha Mishra.
Published/Produced	Hershey, PA: IGI Global, Medical Information Science Reference, [2020]
Description	1 online resource
ISBN	9781799825258 (ebook) (hardcover)
LC classification	SB305
Related names	Mishra, Neha, 1984- editor.
Summary	""This book explores the biosynthesis, phytochemistry, and pharmacology of Indian spices"--Provided by publisher.
Contents	Phytochemistry and pharmacological properties of Zingiber officinale essential oil and extracts: Phytochemistry and Pharmacology of Ginger essential oil and extracts -- Pharmacology and Phytochemistry of Coriander -- Phytochemistry and Ethanopharmacology of IlliciumVerum (Star anise): Ethanopharmacology of llicium Verum -- Spices - Pharmacological and Anti-diabetic activities: Introduction Diabetes Mellitus Mechanism of glucose homeostasis, Anti-diabetic spices & their dosage -- Importance of pest and pathogen control system with special emphasis on coriander crop in Indian subcontinent: Coriander: How to manage pests and pathogens -- Pharmacological activity and Nutritional Potential of Buchanania lanzan Spreng -- Nano Approach - Spices as Antimicrobial Agent -- Pharmacological and Phytochemical Properties of

	Garlic -- Potential health benefits of Fenugreek with multiple pharmacological properties -- Saffron-The king of Spices -- Turmeric: Biological operations and medicinal applications
Subjects	Spices
	Ethnopharmacology--methods
	Plant, Medicinal--chemistry
	India
Notes	Includes bibliographical references and index.
	Description based on print version record and CIP data provided by publisher.
Additional formats	Print version: Ethnopharmacological investigation of Indian spices Hershey, PA: Medical Information Science Reference, [2020] 9781799825241 (DLC) 2019040958

Ethnopharmacological investigation of Indian spices

LCCN	2019040958
Type of material	Book
Main title	Ethnopharmacological investigation of Indian spices / Neha Mishra.
Published/Produced	Hershey, PA: Medical Information Science Reference, [2020]
Description	xx, 335 pages; 29 cm
ISBN	9781799825241 (hardcover)
	(ebook)
LC classification	SB305 .E94 2020
Related names	Mishra, Neha, 1984- editor.
Summary	""This book explores the biosynthesis, phytochemistry, and pharmacology of Indian spices"--Provided by publisher.
Contents	Phytochemistry and pharmacological properties of Zingiber officinale essential oil and extracts: Phytochemistry and Pharmacology of Ginger essential oil and extracts -- Pharmacology and Phytochemistry of Coriander -- Phytochemistry and Ethanopharmacology of IlliciumVerum (Star anise): Ethanopharmacology of Ilicium Verum -- Spices - Pharmacological and Anti-diabetic activities:

Bibliography 85

	Introduction Diabetes Mellitus Mechanism of glucose homeostasis, Anti-diabetic spices & their dosage -- Importance of pest and pathogen control system with special emphasis on coriander crop in Indian subcontinent: Coriander: How to manage pests and pathogens -- Pharmacological activity and Nutritional Potential of Buchanania lanzan Spreng -- Nano Approach - Spices as Antimicrobial Agent -- Pharmacological and Phytochemical Properties of Garlic -- Potential health benefits of Fenugreek with multiple pharmacological properties -- Saffron-The king of Spices -- Turmeric: Biological operations and medicinal applications
Subjects	Spices
	Ethnopharmacology--methods
	Plant, Medicinal--chemistry
	India
Notes	Includes bibliographical references (pages 269-327) and index.
Additional formats	Online version: Ethnopharmacological investigation of Indian spices Hershey, PA: Medical Information Science Reference, [2020] 9781799825258 (DLC) 2019040959

From garden to glass: 80 botanical beverages made from the finest fruits, cordials, and infusions

LCCN	2018957475
Type of material	Book
Personal name	Hurst, David, author.
Main title	From garden to glass: 80 botanical beverages made from the finest fruits, cordials, and infusions / David Hurst.
Published/Produced	New York, NY: Universe Publishing, 2019.
Description	176 pages: color illustrations; 22 cm
ISBN	9780789336545 (hardcover)
	0789336545 (hardcover)
LC classification	TX815 .H86 2019
Summary	""Garden to glass" recipes for nutrient-packed non-alcoholic infusions and cordials based on fresh from

	the garden or farmstand fruits, berries, herbs, and spices used as restorative tonics or as the basis for healthy cocktails. Organized according to main ingredient, the recipes are created with an eye toward both health and taste. All recipes include fresh from the garden botanicals such as elderberries, strawberries, tomato, mints, and other herbs. Each creation is expertly crafted and inspired by some of the most exciting trends in bartending and mixology. The book also explains how to make professional-quality mixed drinks in your home, listing essential bar kit, fancy glassware, party planning, and finishing touches that can transform an ordinary drink into an exceptional cocktail. Includes ideas about 'how to cocktail your mocktail'"-- Adapted from Amazon.com.
Contents	Alcohol-free enjoyment -- First things first -- Herbs. Elderflower -- Basil -- Mint & Thyme -- Spices. Cardamom -- Ginger -- Vanilla -- Citrus. Orange -- Lemon & Lime -- Grapefruit -- Tropical. Pineapple -- Lychee -- Coconut -- Kiwi -- Avocado and mango -- Berries. Cranberry -- Strawberry & Raspberry -- Blueberries & other berries -- Beans. Cocoa -- Coffee -- Pitcher party.
Subjects	Beverages. Fruit drinks. Non-alcoholic cocktails. Cocktails.
Notes	Originally published in the United Kingdom, Australia and New Zealand in 2019 by Modern Books. Includes index.

Ginger: antioxidant properties, functions and medicinal benefits

LCCN	2020679381
Type of material	Book
Main title	Ginger: antioxidant properties, functions and medicinal benefits / Janine L. Perry, editor.
Published/Produced	New York: Nova Publishers, [2015]

Description	1 online resource
ISBN	9781634820363 (eBook)
LC classification	RM666.G488
Related names	Perry, Janine L.
Subjects	Ginger--Therapeutic use.
	Ginger--Therapeutic use.
Notes	Includes bibliographical references and index.
	Description based on online resource; title from PDF title page (Site, viewed 07/23/2020).
Additional formats	Print version: Ginger New York: Nova Publishers, [2015] 9781634820202 (DLC) 2015930586
Series	Food and beverage consumption and health
	Food and beverage consumption and health series.

Ginger: antioxidant properties, functions and medicinal benefits

LCCN	2015930586
Type of material	Book
Main title	Ginger: antioxidant properties, functions and medicinal benefits / Janine L. Perry, editor.
Published/Produced	New York: Nova Publishers, [2015]
	©2015
Description	x, 154 pages: illustrations; 24 cm.
ISBN	9781634820202
	ebook
	1634820207
LC classification	RM666.G488 G55 2015
Related names	Perry, Janine L.
Subjects	Ginger--Therapeutic use.
	Ginger--Therapeutic use.
Notes	Includes bibliographical references and index.
Series	Food and beverage consumption and health
	Food and beverage consumption and health series.

Growing up gourmet: 125 healthy meals for everybody and every baby

LCCN	2015046385
Type of material	Book
Personal name	Carlson, Jennifer, 1975- author.

Main title	Growing up gourmet: 125 healthy meals for everybody and every baby / Jennifer Carlson; with Jennifer House, MSc, RD.
Edition	First Atria Books hardcover edition.
Published/Produced	New York: Atria Books, [2016]
Description	xi, 228 pages: color illustrations; 20 cm
ISBN	9781501110559 (hardback)
LC classification	RJ216 .C33 2016
Summary	"Garlic, cinnamon, cardamom, sage, basil--you'll be amazed by what your baby will eat! Here are 125 healthy, delicious, kitchen-tested, and pediatric dietician-approved baby food recipes that will nurture your child's adventurous palate and guarantee smiles from everyone at the dinner table. Baby Gourmet is a total guide to your baby and toddler's diet. Jennifer Carlson built her business, Baby Gourmet, into one of the top-selling organic baby food brands in North America--and she'll show you how to make nutritious, delicious, home-cooked meals that will complement your child's development schedule and make everyone else in the family happy too. Her mouth-watering recipes reduce picky eating and introduce your baby to the wide world of textures and tastes, from veggies such as kale and fennel, to grains such as amaranth and spelt, to herbs and spices such as turmeric and ginger that will help you avoid added sugar, salt, colorings, and preservatives. As a busy mother of two, Jen understands that it's easy to feel overwhelmed by feeding struggles and the sheer mass of parenting information, not to mention the challenges of finding time to make wholesome, flavorful meals from scratch. In this essential guide, she clearly lays out everything you need to know about feeding your baby: when to wean; how to get the right nutrients at every stage; how to deal with finicky eating habits; which foods will treat gassiness, colic, constipation, low iron, or poor sleep; and how to adapt your special dietary considerations for your child. As

	daunting as it may seem, there are shortcuts and techniques to make it all manageable, whether you're cooking for a single little one or a family of five and counting"-- Provided by publisher.
Subjects	Infants--Nutrition.
	Toddlers--Nutrition.
	Baby foods.
	Cooking / Baby Food.
	Cooking / Specific Ingredients / Natural Foods.
	Cooking / Health & Healing / Allergy.
Additional formats	Online version: Carlson, Jennifer, 1975- author. Growing up gourmet First Atria Books hardcover edition. New York: Atria Books, [2016] 9781501110566 (DLC) 2015046951

Gut health hacks: 200 ways to balance your gut microbiome and improve your health!

LCCN	2021007343
Type of material	Book
Personal name	Boyers, Lindsay, author.
Main title	Gut health hacks: 200 ways to balance your gut microbiome and improve your health! / Lindsay Boyers, CHNC; with a technical review by Murdoc Khaleg, MD.
Edition	First Adams Media trade paperback edition.
Published/Produced	New York: Adams Media, 2021.
Projected pub date	2107
Description	pages cm.
ISBN	9781507216453 (trade paperback)
	(ebook)
LC classification	RC806 .B693 2021
Summary	"Bloating. Heartburn. Weight gain. Frequent visits to the restroom. It's no surprise: bad gut health can have a big impact on your daily life. But what if there were quick and easy ways to improve your digestive system so you could feel your best every day? In Gut Health Hacks, you'll find 200 practical tips and tricks to support good bacteria and achieve a balanced gut mircrobiome. From ways to hack

your meals to simple lifestyle changes, you'll find tips and tricks like: consuming ginger has a calming sensation for your digestive tract and can relieve gas and bloating; sipping some ginger tea before bedtime can lead to a restful night's sleep; mental stress leads to digestive stress; and much more! From improved mental health to weight loss to resolved digestion issues, balanced gut health can make all the difference. Now you can start feeling your best today with a little help from Gut Health Hacks"-- Provided by publisher.

Subjects	Gastrointestinal system--Diseases--Diet therapy.
	Nutrition.
	Self-care, Health--Popular works.
Notes	Includes index.
Series	Hacks

Healing smoothies: 100 research-based, delicious recipes that provide nutrition support for cancer prevention and recovery

LCCN	2015002827
Type of material	Book
Personal name	Chace, Daniella.
Main title	Healing smoothies: 100 research-based, delicious recipes that provide nutrition support for cancer prevention and recovery / Daniella Chace, MSc, CN.
Published/Produced	New York, NY: Skyhorse Publishing, [2015]
Description	232 pages: color illustrations; 20 x 20 cm
ISBN	9781632204479 (hardback)
LC classification	RC271.D52 C525 2015
Summary	"100 Research-Based, Delicious Recipes That Provide Nutrition Support for Prevention and Recovery Fight cancer and help prevent recurrence with these delicious smoothies! Over the last few years there has been a tremendous surge in research identifying the specific nutrients that have the ability to change the course of cancer. With a clearer understanding of the role that food nutrients, toxins, and microflora play in disease prevention and development, we have some of the long sought

answers to our questions about what triggers, promotes, heals, and prevents cancer. Chace offers medicinally-potent smoothie recipes that taste great and provide cancer protective and healing nutrients, such as: Banana Coconut Cocoa Cream Banana Ginger Dream Basil Berry Citrus Carotenoid Crush Cherry Berry Lime Creamy Citrus Berry Kumquat Berry Cherry Tangerine Currant Citrus Watermelon Blackberry and Ginger And many more! The ingredients section of the book provides more than sixty cancer-healing foods that are perfect smoothie additions. Cancer patients and their care providers can use these smoothie recipes or create their own from the ingredients list to help heal and nourish the patient throughout the treatment process. In addition, many of the nutrients in these smoothies have been found to support remission and reduce the risk for cancer recurrence"-- Provided by publisher. "Over the last few years there has been a tremendous surge in research identifying the specific nutrients that have the ability to change the course of cancer. With a clearer understanding of the role that food nutrients, toxins, and microflora play in disease prevention and development, we have some of the long sought answers to our questions about what triggers, promotes, heals, and prevents cancer. Chace offers medicinally-potent smoothie recipes that taste great and provide cancer protective and healing nutrients, such as: Banana Coconut Cocoa Cream Banana Ginger Dream Basil Berry Citrus Carotenoid Crush Cherry Berry Lime Creamy Citrus Berry Kumquat Berry Cherry Tangerine Currant Citrus Watermelon Blackberry and Ginger And many more! The ingredients section of the book provides more than sixty cancer-healing foods that are perfect smoothie additions. Cancer patients and their care providers can use these smoothie recipes or create their own from the ingredients list to help heal and nourish the patient throughout the treatment

	process. In addition, many of the nutrients in these smoothies have been found to support remission and reduce the risk for cancer recurrence"-- Provided by publisher.
Subjects	Cancer--Diet therapy--Recipes.
	Cancer--Nutritional aspects.
	Smoothies (Beverages)
	Health & Fitness / Diseases / Cancer.
Form/Genre	Cookbooks.
Notes	Includes bibliographical references and index.

Healthcare in motion: immobilities in health service delivery and access

LCCN	2018018667
Type of material	Book
Main title	Healthcare in motion: immobilities in health service delivery and access / edited by Cecilia Vindrola-Padros, Ginger A. Johnson, and Anne E. Pfister.
Published/Produced	New York: Berghahn Books, 2018.
Projected pub date	1808
Description	1 online resource.
ISBN	9781785339547 (ebook)
LC classification	RA393
Related names	Vindrola-Padros, Cecilia, 1983- editor.
Subjects	Health services accessibility.
	Health planning.
	Medical policy--Social aspects.
	Minorities--Medical care.
Notes	Includes bibliographical references and index.
	Description based on print version record and CIP data provided by publisher; resource not viewed.
Additional formats	Print version: Healthcare in motion New York: Berghahn Books, 2018 9781785339530 (DLC) 2018006185
Series	Worlds in motion; volume 5

Healthcare in motion: immobilities in health service delivery and access

LCCN	2018006185
Type of material	Book

Main title	Healthcare in motion: immobilities in health service delivery and access / edited by Cecilia Vindrola-Padros, Ginger A. Johnson, and Anne E. Pfister.
Published/Produced	New York: Berghahn Books, 2018.
Description	viii, 232 pages; 24 cm.
ISBN	9781785339530 (hardback: alk. paper)
	1785339532 (hardback: alk. paper)
LC classification	RA393 .H3746 2018
Related names	Vindrola-Padros, Cecilia, 1983- editor.
Subjects	Health services accessibility.
	Health planning.
	Medical policy--Social aspects.
	Minorities--Medical care.
Notes	Includes bibliographical references and index.
Additional formats	Online version: Healthcare in motion New York: Berghahn Books, 2018 9781785339547 (DLC) 2018018667
Series	Worlds in motion; volume 5

Healthy one pan dinners: 100 easy recipes for your sheet pan, skillet, multicooker, and more

LCCN	2019950714
Type of material	Book
Personal name	White, Dana Angelo, author.
Main title	Healthy one pan dinners: 100 easy recipes for your sheet pan, skillet, multicooker, and more / Dana Angelo White, MS, RD, ATC.
Edition	First American edition.
Published/Produced	Indianapolis, Indiana: DK Publishing, 2020. ©2020
Description	159 pages: color illustrations; 24 cm
ISBN	9781465492661 (paperback)
	1465492666 (paperback)
LC classification	TX833.5 .W4923 2020
Variant title	Healthy 1 pan dinners: one hundred easy recipes for your sheet pan, skillet, multicooker, and more
Related names	Schuyler, Kelley Jordan, photographer.
Summary	Ditch the dishes and simplify dinner with 100 healthy, family-friendly recipes you can make in just

one pan. Weeknight dinners can be a chore, especially when they require multiple pots and pans. Simplify dinner with 100 easy recipes that come together quickly and require only one sheet pan, skillet, Dutch oven, multicooker, or slow cooker. Healthy recipes feature fresh, whole food ingredients and lightened up versions of family favorites. Short on prep but big on flavor, these homemade meals are easy, flexible, and quick to prepare--exactly what you need to get dinner on the table with minimal fuss. Healthy One Pan Dinners makes weeknight cooking attainable with: - 100 recipes for satisfying, one-pan dinners that will please the whole family including Skirt Steak with Chimichurri, Ginger Shrimp with Carrots and Snap Peas, Eggplant Parmesan Stackers, and Thai Chicken Lettuce Cups. - Helpful tags to identify Gluten-Free, Dairy-Free, Vegetarian, Under 30 Minutes, and Freezer-Friendly meals. - Complete nutritional information for every recipe. - Tips for repurposing leftovers, meal prep, storage, and reheating.

Contents Introduction -- The healthy one pan kitchen -- Sheet pan -- Skillet -- Dutch oven -- Baking dish -- Multicooker + slow cooker

Subjects Quick and easy cooking.
One-dish meals.
Low-fat diet--Recipes.
Low-calorie diet--Recipes.
Cooking / Health & Healing / Low Fat.
Cooking / Health & Healing / Weight Control.
Cooking / Methods / Quick & Easy.
Low-calorie diet.
Low-fat diet.
One-dish meals.
Quick and easy cooking.

Form/Genre Cookbooks.
Recipes.
Cookbooks.

Notes	Cookbooks. Includes index.

Home remedies: how to use kitchen staples to cure common ailments

LCCN	2019029175
Type of material	Book
Personal name	Bruton-Seal, Julie, author.
Uniform title	Kitchen medicine
Main title	Home remedies: how to use kitchen staples to cure common ailments / Julie Bruton-Seal, Matthew Seal.
Published/Produced	New York City: Skyhorse Publishing, [2019]
ISBN	9781510754065 (ebook) (paperback)
LC classification	RC82
Related names	Seal, Matthew, 1946- author.
Summary	"A complete herbal handbook of home cures and kitchen remedies from the team behind Backyard Medicine and Backyard Medicine for All. Years ago, every household practiced kitchen medicine. Doctors were expensive and people were self-reliant-even when it came to health care. Today, doctors are more expensive and we've become much less self-reliant. Now Home Remedies revives that lost tradition of the kitchen as pharmacy. Learn how: Fennel wards off symptoms of menopause Garlic reduces cholesterol levels Lemon relieves rheumatism Ginger treats a cold An olive oil purge can eliminate gallstones Sore joints are eased with mustard So much more! With great original photography, foolproof recipes, and fascinating insights into the history of these household ingredients, Home Remedies gives you the "medicinal intelligence" to create your own remedies and cures from the remarkable treasures found sitting in your kitchen right now"-- Provided by publisher.
Subjects	Medicine, Popular. Traditional medicine.

Notes	Kitchens. "Originally published as Kitchen medicine in the United Kingdom by Merlin Unwin Books Limited."--Title page verso. Includes bibliographical references and index. Description based on print version record and CIP data provided by publisher; resource not viewed.
Additional formats	Print version: Bruton-Seal, Julie. Home remedies New York City: Skyhorse Publishing, [2019] 9781510754058 (DLC) 2019029174
Series	Backyard medicine

Home remedies: how to use kitchen staples to cure common ailments

LCCN	2019029174
Type of material	Book
Personal name	Bruton-Seal, Julie, author.
Uniform title	Kitchen medicine
Main title	Home remedies: how to use kitchen staples to cure common ailments / Julie Bruton-Seal, Matthew Seal.
Published/Produced	New York City: Skyhorse Publishing, [2019]
ISBN	9781510754058 (paperback) (ebook)
LC classification	RC82 .B785 2019
Related names	Seal, Matthew, 1946- author.
Summary	"A complete herbal handbook of home cures and kitchen remedies from the team behind Backyard Medicine and Backyard Medicine for All. Years ago, every household practiced kitchen medicine. Doctors were expensive and people were self-reliant-even when it came to health care. Today, doctors are more expensive and we've become much less self-reliant. Now Home Remedies revives that lost tradition of the kitchen as pharmacy. Learn how: Fennel wards off symptoms of menopause Garlic reduces cholesterol levels Lemon relieves rheumatism Ginger treats a cold An olive oil purge can eliminate gallstones Sore joints are eased with mustard So much more! With great original

photography, foolproof recipes, and fascinating insights into the history of these household ingredients, Home Remedies gives you the "medicinal intelligence" to create your own remedies and cures from the remarkable treasures found sitting in your kitchen right now"-- Provided by publisher.

Subjects	Medicine, Popular.
	Traditional medicine.
	Kitchens.
Notes	"Originally published as Kitchen medicine in the United Kingdom by Merlin Unwin Books Limited."--Title page verso.
	Includes bibliographical references and index.
Additional formats	Online version: Bruton-Seal, Julie, Home remedies New York City: Skyhorse Publishing, 2019. 9781510754065 (DLC) 2019029175
Series	Backyard medicine

Infusing flavors: recipes for oils, vinegars, sauces, bitters, waters & more

LCCN	2015047474
Type of material	Book
Personal name	Coopey, Erin, author.
Main title	Infusing flavors: recipes for oils, vinegars, sauces, bitters, waters & more / Erin Coopey.
Published/Produced	Minneapolis, Minnesota: Cool Springs Press, 2016.
Description	176 pages: illustrations; 24 cm
ISBN	9781591866541 (paperback)
LC classification	TX819.A1 C6548 2016
Summary	"Ready to escape "vanilla" ho-hum recipes, embrace your culinary creativity, and taste something new? Yeah, we thought so. Pick up this cookbook--your ticket to a world of flavor.Infusing Flavors features recipes to infuse mind-blowing flavors into teas, tisanes, bitters, liqueurs, aguas frescas, waters, vinegars, oils, gastriques, shrubs, ice creams, soft drinks, and more. Each section in the book is packed with unique recipes. You'll learn which herbs, fruits, flowers, vegetables, and even seeds can be prepared

and infused into all-natural food and drink recipes. With its emphasis on flavor infusions that stretch beyond your standard cocktail bitters, this book is a special treat for any food lover.Here's a taste of some of the ingredients you'll use in Infusing Flavors:Herbs and flowers - chamomile, lavender, lemongrass, rosemary, mint, sage, thyme, lemon verbena, ginger, basilFruits - cherry, peach, strawberries, raspberries, blackberries, blueberries, citrus (lemons and oranges), watermelonVeggies, berries, and roots - celery, fennel, dandelionThe blending and infusing chapter, plus the diverse recipe sections of the cookbook, promise to keep readers enthralled and learning something they never guessed about these wide-ranging ingredients for flavor infusion. The book includes information about the following:Peel-to-stem is the new nose-to-tail: introduction to the movement Blending Infusing Storing Experimenting with flavors Health benefits (including tips on growing your own fresh herbs)The RecipesTeas and tisanes - herbal and fruit; iced and hotHoneys, sugars, and simple syrupsExtracts and bitters - from baker to bartenderShrubs, switchels, and kombuchasSoft drinks and infused waters (sodas, beer, and "ade")Flavored oils - the chef's secretVinegars and gastriquesBrothsDesserts and sweets"-- Provided by publisher.

Subjects Cooking (Spices)
Herbal teas.
Flavoring essences.
Essences and essential oils.
Non-alcoholic beverages--Flavor and odor.
Oils and fats--Flavor and odor.
Cooking / Beverages / General.
Cooking / Methods / General.
Cooking / Specific Ingredients / Herbs, Spices, Condiments.

Form/Genre Cookbooks.

Bibliography 99

Notes	Includes index.

Korean functional foods: composition, processing, and health benefits

LCCN	2017045664
Type of material	Book
Main title	Korean functional foods: composition, processing, and health benefits / edited by Kun-Young Park, Dae Young Kwon, Ki Won Lee, Sunmin Park.
Published/Produced	Boca Raton: CRC Press, Taylor & Francis Group, [2018]
Description	xx, 564 pages: illustrations, maps; 24 cm.
ISBN	9781498799652 (hardback: acid-free paper)
LC classification	QP144.F85 K6745 2018
Related names	Pak, Kŏn-yŏng (Professor of food and nutrition), editor. Kwon, Dae Young, editor. Lee, Ki Won, editor. Park, Sunmin, editor.
Summary	Koreans believe the adage of food as medicine. Therefore, herbs or fruit ingredients such as ginger, cinnamon, adlay, mugwort, pomegranate, and ginseng are used for their therapeutic effects as much as cooking. This book provide information related to Korean functional food. It first describes the history and culture of Korean foods, and then compares Korean diet tables with other Asian countries and Western countries. Also, the book will cover detailed information of Korean functional foods such as kimchi, soybean products, ginseng, salt, oil and seeds. It also deals with its health benefits and processing methods, followed by rules and regulations related to its manufacture and sales. -- Provided by publisher.
Subjects	Functional foods. Cooking, Korean. Diet therapy.
Notes	Includes bibliographical references and index.
Series	Functional foods and nutraceuticals series

Magic soup: 100 recipes for health and happiness

LCCN	2015510810
Type of material	Book
Personal name	Pisani, Nicole, author.
Main title	Magic soup: 100 recipes for health and happiness / Nicole Pisani and Kate Adams.
Edition	First Atria Books hardcover edition.
Published/Produced	New York: Atria Books, 2015.
Description	239 pages: color illustrations; 26 cm
Links	Contributor biographical information http://www.loc.gov/catdir/enhancements/fy1605/2015510810-b.html
	Publisher description http://www.loc.gov/catdir/enhancements/fy1605/2015510810-d.html
	Sample text http://www.loc.gov/catdir/enhancements/fy1605/2015510810-s.html
ISBN	1501127136
	9781501127137
LC classification	TX757 .P57 2015
Related names	Adams, Kate (Health publisher), author.
Summary	"Magic Soup is a mouth-watering collection of more than one hundred innovative recipes for stocks and stews, hearty meals, healing bone broths, a detoxifying soup cleanse, and more. Recipes such as salmon poached in lemongrass tea, lemon chicken and mint with quinoa, and the ultimate "chicken soup for the soul" prove that soup can be a filling meal in itself. There's drool-worthy butternut squash with caramelized pear; delicious beetroot and burrata; and a robust Swedish sailors' soup made from beef and beer. In warmer months, cool down with watermelon gazpacho and fennel vichyssoise. And get healthy with nettle soup with flowers, a miso soup for each season, and the book's namesake restorative magic soup of turmeric, ginger, cardamom, cayenne, cinnamon, cumin, spinach, and seeds,"--Amazon.com.
Contents	Introduction -- Soup Essentials -- Stocks -- Quick Fixes -- Roots & Tubers -- Cleansing -- Old Wives'

	Tales -- Around The World -- Comfort -- Feasts -- Chilled -- On The Side -- Favorite Recipe Books & Journals -- Index -- About Kate & Nicole -- Acknowledgments.
Subjects	Soups.
	Reducing diets.
Notes	Includes bibliographical references (page 230) and index.

Medicinal plants: bioprospecting and pharmacognosy

LCCN	2021060275
Type of material	Book
Main title	Medicinal plants: bioprospecting and pharmacognosy / edited by Amit Baran Sharangi, K. V. Peter.
Edition	First edition.
Published/Produced	Palm Bay, FL, USA: Apple Academic Press, 2022.
Description	1 online resource
ISBN	9781003277408 (ebook)
	(hardback)
	(paperback)
LC classification	RS431.M37
Related names	Sharangi, A. B. (Amit Baran), editor.
	Peter, K. V., editor.
Summary	"With chapters written by scientists from respected institutes and universities around the world, this book looks at the bioprospecting of medicinal plants for potential health uses and at the pharmacognosy of a selection of medicinal and aromatic plants. The book touches on a diverse selection of topics related to medicinal plants. Chapters look at the use of medicinal plants in healthcare and disease management, such as to treat inflammation, anti-hyperglycemia, and obesity and as immunity boosters. The authors also address the conservation, maintenance, and sustainable utilization of medicinal plants along with postharvest management issues. A chapter discusses the use of synthetic seeds in relation to cryopreservation, and a

Bibliography

Contents

chapter is devoted to the use of microcomputed tomography and image processing tools in medicinal and aromatic plants. Other topics include consumption, supply chain, marketing, trade, and future directions of research. Some specific plants discussed include fennel, basil, clove, ginger, lavender, turmeric, ginsing, and asparagus in connection with their various therapeutic properties, including anti-rheumatic, anti-asthmatic, anti-diabetic, carminative, diuretic, fever-reducing, and hypotensive. Medicinal Plants: Bioprospecting and Pharmacognosy will prove informative for scientists and researchers in medicinal plants as well as for faculty and students, pharmaceutical researchers, and others"-- Provided by publisher.

1. Medicinal plants: perspectives and retrospectives 2. Traditional medicine in health care and disease management 3. Herbal drug discovery against inflammation: from traditional wisdom to modern therapeutics 4. Foeniculum vulgare mill: flavoring, pharmacological, phytochemical, and folklore aspects 5. Ocimum basilicum: a model medicinal industrial crop enriched with an array of bioactive chemicals 6. Syzygium aromaticum, curcuma longa, and lavandula: volatile components and antioxidant activities 7. Anti-hyperglycemic property of medicinal plants 8. Improved production and postharvest technologies in ashwagandha (Indian ginseng) 9. Endangered medicinal plants of temperate regions: conservation and maintenance 10. Conservation and sustainable utilization of threatened medicinal plants of North East India 11. Essential oils: clinical perspectives and uses 12. Asparagus sp.: phytochemicals and marketed herbal formulations 13. Phytosomes: preparations, characterization, and future uses 14. Synthetic seeds vis a vis cryopreservation: an efficient technique for long-term preservation of endangered medicinal plants 15. Use of microcomputed tomography and

	image processing tools in medicinal and aromatic plants 16. Postharvest care of medicinal and aromatic plants: a reservoir of many health benefiting constituents 17. Prosopis cineraria (khejri): ethanopharmacology and phytochemistry 18. Mitigation of obesity: a phytotherapeutic approach 19. Ethnomedicinal plants of North Eastern Himalayan region of India to combat hypertension 20. Medicinal plants: consumption, supply chain, marketing, and trade in India 21. Potential of spices as medicines and immunity boosters 22. Medicinal plants: future thrust areas and research directions.
Subjects	Medicinal plants.
	Materia medica, Vegetable.
	Pharmacognosy.
	Botanical drug industry.
Notes	Includes bibliographical references and index.
	Description based on print version record and CIP data provided by publisher; resource not viewed.
Additional formats	Also available online.
	Print version: Medicinal plants First edition. Palm Bay, FL, USA: Apple Academic Press, 2022 9781774638453 (DLC) 2021060274
Series	Innovations in horticultural science
	Innovations in horticultural science.

Medicinal plants: bioprospecting and pharmacognosy

LCCN	2021060274
Type of material	Book
Main title	Medicinal plants: bioprospecting and pharmacognosy / edited by Amit Baran Sharangi, K. V. Peter.
Edition	First edition.
Published/Produced	Palm Bay, FL, USA: Apple Academic Press, 2022.
ISBN	9781774638453 (hardback)
	9781774638460 (paperback)
	(ebook)
LC classification	RS431.M37 M44 2022

Bibliography

Related names	Sharangi, A. B. (Amit Baran), editor.
	Peter, K. V., editor.
Summary	"With chapters written by scientists from respected institutes and universities around the world, this book looks at the bioprospecting of medicinal plants for potential health uses and at the pharmacognosy of a selection of medicinal and aromatic plants. The book touches on a diverse selection of topics related to medicinal plants. Chapters look at the use of medicinal plants in healthcare and disease management, such as to treat inflammation, anti-hyperglycemia, and obesity and as immunity boosters. The authors also address the conservation, maintenance, and sustainable utilization of medicinal plants along with postharvest management issues. A chapter discusses the use of synthetic seeds in relation to cryopreservation, and a chapter is devoted to the use of microcomputed tomography and image processing tools in medicinal and aromatic plants. Other topics include consumption, supply chain, marketing, trade, and future directions of research. Some specific plants discussed include fennel, basil, clove, ginger, lavender, turmeric, ginsing, and asparagus in connection with their various therapeutic properties, including anti-rheumatic, anti-asthmatic, anti-diabetic, carminative, diuretic, fever-reducing, and hypotensive. Medicinal Plants: Bioprospecting and Pharmacognosy will prove informative for scientists and researchers in medicinal plants as well as for faculty and students, pharmaceutical researchers, and others"-- Provided by publisher.
Contents	1. Medicinal plants: perspectives and retrospectives 2. Traditional medicine in health care and disease management 3. Herbal drug discovery against inflammation: from traditional wisdom to modern therapeutics 4. Foeniculum vulgare mill: flavoring, pharmacological, phytochemical, and folklore aspects 5. Ocimum basilicum: a model medicinal

industrial crop enriched with an array of bioactive chemicals 6. Syzygium aromaticum, curcuma longa, and lavandula: volatile components and antioxidant activities 7. Anti-hyperglycemic property of medicinal plants 8. Improved production and postharvest technologies in ashwagandha (Indian ginseng) 9. Endangered medicinal plants of temperate regions: conservation and maintenance 10. Conservation and sustainable utilization of threatened medicinal plants of North East India 11. Essential oils: clinical perspectives and uses 12. Asparagus sp.: phytochemicals and marketed herbal formulations 13. Phytosomes: preparations, characterization, and future uses 14. Synthetic seeds vis a vis cryopreservation: an efficient technique for long-term preservation of endangered medicinal plants 15. Use of microcomputed tomography and image processing tools in medicinal and aromatic plants 16. Postharvest care of medicinal and aromatic plants: a reservoir of many health benefiting constituents 17. Prosopis cineraria (khejri): ethanopharmacology and phytochemistry 18. Mitigation of obesity: a phytotherapeutic approach 19. Ethnomedicinal plants of North Eastern Himalayan region of India to combat hypertension 20. Medicinal plants: consumption, supply chain, marketing, and trade in India 21. Potential of spices as medicines and immunity boosters 22. Medicinal plants: future thrust areas and research directions.

Subjects Medicinal plants.
Materia medica, Vegetable.
Pharmacognosy.
Botanical drug industry.

Notes Includes bibliographical references and index.
Additional formats Also available online.
Online version: Medicinal plants First edition. Palm Bay, FL, USA: Apple Academic Press, 2022 9781003277408 (DLC) 2021060275

Meet your matcha: over 50 irresistible recipes packed with the power of green tea

Series	Innovations in horticultural science Innovations in horticultural science.
LCCN	2017297145
Type of material	Book
Personal name	Farrow, Joanna.
Main title	Meet your matcha: over 50 irresistible recipes packed with the power of green tea / Joanna Farrow.
Published/Produced	London: Nourish, 2017.
Description	111 pages: colour illustrations; 20 cm
ISBN	1848993404 9781848993402
LC classification	TX817.T3 F37 2017
Portion of title	Over 50 irresistible recipes packed with the power of green tea
Summary	"Matcha teas and lattes have become a staple of every coffee shop and health food store. A beloved ingredient in Japan for generations, it is a powdered green tea that is rich in nutrients and antioxidants, and gives a slow-release caffeine boost through the day. One glass of matcha is the equivalent of 10 glasses of green tea in terms of nutritional value and antioxidant content. But there is so much more you can do with this miracle ingredient. Packed with over 50 recipes for smoothies, soups, main meals and more, Meet Your Matcha will allow you to unlock the potential of this brilliant green ingredient. From a Matcha Sushi Salad and Matcha Chicken and Ginger Dumplings to Breakfast Smoothie Bowls or a Dark Chocolate and Matcha Layer Cake, these delicious dishes will let you make the most of your matcha." -- Provided by publisher.
Contents	Smoothies & breakfasts -- Main meals -- Salads & sides -- Desserts & cakes -- Sweet treats -- Teas, juices & cocktails.
Subjects	Cooking (Tea) Green tea.

	Illustrated books.
	Cooking (Tea)
	Green tea.
	Illustrated books.
Form/Genre	Cookbooks.
	Cookbooks.
Notes	Includes index.

Natural medicine for horses: home remedies and natural healing

LCCN	2016304802
Type of material	Book
Personal name	Wittek, Cornelia, author.
Uniform title	Von Apfelessig bis Teebaumöl. English
Main title	Natural medicine for horses: home remedies and natural healing / Cornelia Wittek; translated by John Kinory.
Published/Produced	Sheffield, U.K: 5M Publishing, 2016. ©2011
Description	xii, 196 pages: color illustrations; 25 cm.
ISBN	9781910455104 (pbk.) 1910455105 (pbk.)
LC classification	SF951 .W5813 2016
Related names	Kinory, John translator.
Summary	Healthy foods, supplements, preparations and remedies based on natural ingredients are increasingly promoted in human health, and can equally be used for your horse's health. Ingredients such as yogurt, ginger and buckwheat can promote general well-being and address specific concerns about equine conditions and ailments. -- Source other than Library of Congress.
Contents	Gentle healp from nature -- Home and natural remedies from a to z -- A varied diet -- Year-round health.
Subjects	Horses--Health.
	Horses--Nutrition--Requirements.
	Horses--Feeding and feeds.
	Horses--Treatment.

Notes	"Copyright ©2011 Franckh-Kosmos Verlags-GmbH & Co., KG, Stuttgart, Germany."--T.p. verso.
	Includes bibliographical references and index.
Series	Horse riding and management series
	Horse riding and management series.

Natural oral care in dental therapy

LCCN	2019050429
Type of material	Book
Main title	Natural oral care in dental therapy / edited by Durgesh Nandini Chauhan, Prabhu Raj Singh, Kamal Shah and Nagendra Singh Chauhan.
Published/Produced	Hoboken, New Jersey: Wiley-Scrivener, [2020]
ISBN	9781119614227 (cloth)
	(adobe pdf)
	(epub)
LC classification	RK305
Related names	Chauhan, Durgesh Nandini, editor.
	Singh, Prabhu Raj, editor.
	Shah, Kamal, editor.
	Chauhan, Nagendra Singh, editor.
Summary	"Patients increasingly seek integrated and anticipatory approaches to their healthcare. In this altering health environment, oral healthcare specialists can influence and expand their long-standing commitment to the preventative care model. Nowadays oral care specialists need to increasingly focus on the interdisciplinary connections between oral health, heart health, gastrointestinal health, etc. This important new volume will be valuable to Principal Dentists, Oral Hygienists, pharmacognosy expert, Natural product formulation scientist alike, either as a textbook or as a reference. It is a must-have for any dentist library and Herbal industry. Discusses natural products that can be used to treat oral diseases and their scientific basis for how these natural product act. Natural products for oral health care are on the increase worldwide and this is the first book to cover all the

Bibliography

Contents

herbal antibiotics. The 26 chapters in this unique book explore all the measures to utilize the natural oral care obtained from plants, animals and mineral drugs for dental care"-- Provided by publisher.

Natural Oral Care in Dental Therapy: Current and Future Prospects / Durgesh Nandini Chauhan, Prabhu Raj Singh, Kamal Shah and Nagendra Singh Chauhan -- Herbal Products for Oral Hygiene: An Overview of Their Biological Activities / Ummuhan Sebnem Harput -- Go Green-Periodontal Care in the Natural Way / Siddhartha Varma and Sameer Anil Zope -- Role of Herbal and Natural Products in the Management of Potentially Malignant Oral Disorders / P Kalyana Chakravarthy, Komal Smriti and Sravan Kumar Yeturu -- Studies on the Anticariogenic Potential of Medicinal Plant Seed and Fruit Extracts / Disha M Patel, Jenabhai B Chauhan and Kalpesh B Ishnava -- Cytotoxic and Anti-Inflammatory Effect of Turmeric and Aloe Vera in a Gingivitis Model / Karen Esperanza Almanza-Aranda, Miguel Aranda-Fonseca, Gabriela Velazquez-Plascencia and Rene Garcia-Contreras -- Effects of Bauhinia forficata Link in Reducing Streptococcus mutans Biofilm on Teeth / Julio Cesar C. Ferreira-Filho, Andressa Temperini de Oliveira Marre, Juliana Soares de Sá Almeida, Leandro de Araújo Lobo, Adriano Gomes Cruz, Marlon Máximo de Andrade, Thiago Isidro Vieira, Maria Teresa Villela Romanos, Mariana Leonel Martins, Lucianne Cople Maia, Ana Maria Gondim Valença and Andréa Fonseca-Gonçalves -- Antimicrobial Effect of a Cardamom Ethanolic Extract on Oral Biofilm: An Ex Vivo Study / Marina Fernandes Binimeliz, Mariana Leonel Martins, Julio Cesar Campos Ferreira Filho, Lucio Mendes Cabral, Adriano Gomes da Cruz, Lucianne Cople Maia and Andréa Fonseca-Gonçalves -- Effect of Punica granatum Peel Extract on Growth of Candida albicans in Oral Mucosa of Diabetic Male Rats /

Maryam Eidi and Fatemeh Noorbakhsh -- Effect of Oil Pulling on Oral Health / Sameer Anil Zope and Siddhartha Varma -- Role of Proteolytic Enzymes in Dental Care / P Kalyana Chakravarthy and Sravan Kumar Yeturu -- The Effect of Probiotic on Oral Health / Patricia Nadelman, Marcela Baraúna Magno, Mariana Farias da Cruz, Adriano Gomes da Cruz, Matheus Melo Pithon, Andréa Fonseca-Gonçalves and Lucianne Cople Maia -- Charcoal in Dentistry / Abhilasha Thakur, Aditya Ganeshpurkar and Anupam Jaiswal -- Propolis Benefits in Oral Health / Mariana Leonel Martins, Karla Lorene de França Leite, Yuri Wanderley Cavalcanti, Lucianne Cople Maia and Andréa Fonseca-Gonçalves -- Grape Seed Extract in Dental Therapy / Anusuya V, Ashok Kumar Jen and Jitendra Sharan -- Ocimum Sanctum L: Promising Agent for Oral Health Care Management / Trinette Fernandes, Anisha D'souza and Sujata P. Sawarkar -- Coconut Palm (Cocos nucifera L.): A Natural Gift to Human Being for Dental Ministrations / Navneet Kishore and Akhilesh Kumar Verma -- Salvadora persica L. (Miswak): An Effective Folklore Toothbrush / Sujata P. Sawarkar, Anisha D'souza and Trinette Fernandes -- Triphala and Oral Health / Kamal Shigli, Sushma S Nayak, Mrinal Shete, Vasanti Lagali Jirge and Veerendra Nanjwade -- Azadirachta indica (Neem): An Ancient Indian Boon to the Contemporary World of Dentistry / Sri Chandana Tanguturi, Sumanth Gunupati and Sreenivas Nagarakanti -- Ginger in Oral Care / Aditya Ganeshpurkar, Abhilasha Thakur and Anupam Jaiswal -- Effectiveness of Allium sativum on Bacterial Oral Infection / Vesna Karic, Jaiswal Anupam, Heidi Abrahamse, Thakur Abhilasha and Ganeshpurkar Aditya -- Curative Plants Worn in the Healing of Mouth Evils / P. Shivakumar Singh, Pindi Pavan Kumar and D. Srinivasulu -- Ethnopharmacological Applications of Chewing

Bibliography

	Sticks on Oral Health Care / Akaji E. A. and Otakhoigbogie U -- Ethnomedicine and Ethnopharmacology for Dental Diseases in Indochina / Viroj Wiwanitkit -- Traditional Medicinal Plants Used in Anti Halitosis / P. Shivakumar Singh, Pindi Pavan Kumar and D. Srinivasulu.
Subjects	Mouth Diseases--drug therapy
	Plants, Medicinal
	Mouth Diseases--prevention & control
	Dental Care
	Medicine, Traditional
Notes	Includes bibliographical references and index.
Additional formats	Online version: Natural oral care in dental therapy Hoboken, New Jersey: Wiley-Scrivener, [2020] 9781119618935 (DLC) 2019050430

Natural oral care in dental therapy

LCCN	2019050430
Type of material	Book
Main title	Natural oral care in dental therapy / edited by Durgesh Nandini Chauhan, Prabhu Raj Singh, Kamal Shah and Nagendra Singh Chauhan.
Published/Produced	Hoboken, New Jersey: Wiley-Scrivener, [2020]
Description	1 online resource
ISBN	9781119618904 (epub)
	9781119618935 (adobe pdf)
	(cloth)
LC classification	RK305
Related names	Chauhan, Durgesh Nandini, editor.
	Singh, Prabhu Raj, editor.
	Shah, Kamal, editor.
	Chauhan, Nagendra Singh, editor.
Summary	"Patients increasingly seek integrated and anticipatory approaches to their healthcare. In this altering health environment, oral healthcare specialists can influence and expand their long-standing commitment to the preventative care model. Nowadays oral care specialists need to

increasingly focus on the interdisciplinary connections between oral health, heart health, gastrointestinal health, etc. This important new volume will be valuable to Principal Dentists, Oral Hygienists, pharmacognosy expert, Natural product formulation scientist alike, either as a textbook or as a reference. It is a must-have for any dentist library and Herbal industry. Discusses natural products that can be used to treat oral diseases and their scientific basis for how these natural product act. Natural products for oral health care are on the increase worldwide and this is the first book to cover all the herbal antibiotics. The 26 chapters in this unique book explore all the measures to utilize the natural oral care obtained from plants, animals and mineral drugs for dental care"-- Provided by publisher.

Contents

Natural Oral Care in Dental Therapy: Current and Future Prospects / Durgesh Nandini Chauhan, Prabhu Raj Singh, Kamal Shah and Nagendra Singh Chauhan -- Herbal Products for Oral Hygiene: An Overview of Their Biological Activities / Ummuhan Sebnem Harput -- Go Green-Periodontal Care in the Natural Way / Siddhartha Varma and Sameer Anil Zope -- Role of Herbal and Natural Products in the Management of Potentially Malignant Oral Disorders / P Kalyana Chakravarthy, Komal Smriti and Sravan Kumar Yeturu -- Studies on the Anticariogenic Potential of Medicinal Plant Seed and Fruit Extracts / Disha M Patel, Jenabhai B Chauhan and Kalpesh B Ishnava -- Cytotoxic and Anti-Inflammatory Effect of Turmeric and Aloe Vera in a Gingivitis Model / Karen Esperanza Almanza-Aranda, Miguel Aranda-Fonseca, Gabriela Velazquez-Plascencia and Rene Garcia-Contreras -- Effects of Bauhinia forficata Link in Reducing Streptococcus mutans Biofilm on Teeth / Julio Cesar C. Ferreira-Filho, Andressa Temperini de Oliveira Marre, Juliana Soares de Sá Almeida, Leandro de Araújo Lobo, Adriano Gomes Cruz,

Marlon Máximo de Andrade, Thiago Isidro Vieira, Maria Teresa Villela Romanos, Mariana Leonel Martins, Lucianne Cople Maia, Ana Maria Gondim Valença and Andréa Fonseca-Gonçalves -- Antimicrobial Effect of a Cardamom Ethanolic Extract on Oral Biofilm: An Ex Vivo Study / Marina Fernandes Binimeliz, Mariana Leonel Martins, Julio Cesar Campos Ferreira Filho, Lucio Mendes Cabral, Adriano Gomes da Cruz, Lucianne Cople Maia and Andréa Fonseca-Gonçalves -- Effect of Punica granatum Peel Extract on Growth of Candida albicans in Oral Mucosa of Diabetic Male Rats / Maryam Eidi and Fatemeh Noorbakhsh -- Effect of Oil Pulling on Oral Health / Sameer Anil Zope and Siddhartha Varma -- Role of Proteolytic Enzymes in Dental Care / P Kalyana Chakravarthy and Sravan Kumar Yeturu -- The Effect of Probiotic on Oral Health / Patricia Nadelman, Marcela Baraúna Magno, Mariana Farias da Cruz, Adriano Gomes da Cruz, Matheus Melo Pithon, Andréa Fonseca-Gonçalves and Lucianne Cople Maia -- Charcoal in Dentistry / Abhilasha Thakur, Aditya Ganeshpurkar and Anupam Jaiswal -- Propolis Benefits in Oral Health / Mariana Leonel Martins, Karla Lorene de França Leite, Yuri Wanderley Cavalcanti, Lucianne Cople Maia and Andréa Fonseca-Gonçalves -- Grape Seed Extract in Dental Therapy / Anusuya V, Ashok Kumar Jen and Jitendra Sharan -- Ocimum Sanctum L: Promising Agent for Oral Health Care Management / Trinette Fernandes, Anisha D'souza and Sujata P. Sawarkar -- Coconut Palm (Cocos nucifera L.): A Natural Gift to Human Being for Dental Ministrations / Navneet Kishore and Akhilesh Kumar Verma -- Salvadora persica L. (Miswak): An Effective Folklore Toothbrush / Sujata P. Sawarkar, Anisha D'souza and Trinette Fernandes -- Triphala and Oral Health / Kamal Shigli, Sushma S Nayak, Mrinal Shete, Vasanti Lagali Jirge and Veerendra Nanjwade --

	Azadirachta indica (Neem): An Ancient Indian Boon to the Contemporary World of Dentistry / Sri Chandana Tanguturi, Sumanth Gunupati and Sreenivas Nagarakanti -- Ginger in Oral Care / Aditya Ganeshpurkar, Abhilasha Thakur and Anupam Jaiswal -- Effectiveness of Allium sativum on Bacterial Oral Infection / Vesna Karic, Jaiswal Anupam, Heidi Abrahamse, Thakur Abhilasha and Ganeshpurkar Aditya -- Curative Plants Worn in the Healing of Mouth Evils / P. Shivakumar Singh, Pindi Pavan Kumar and D. Srinivasulu -- Ethnopharmacological Applications of Chewing Sticks on Oral Health Care / Akaji E. A. and Otakhoigbogie U -- Ethnomedicine and Ethnopharmacology for Dental Diseases in Indochina / Viroj Wiwanitkit -- Traditional Medicinal Plants Used in Anti Halitosis / P. Shivakumar Singh, Pindi Pavan Kumar and D. Srinivasulu.
Subjects	Mouth Diseases--drug therapy
	Plants, Medicinal
	Mouth Diseases--prevention & control
	Dental Care
	Medicine, Traditional
Notes	Includes bibliographical references and index.
	Description based on print version record and CIP data provided by publisher.
Additional formats	Print version: Natural oral care in dental therapy Hoboken, New Jersey: Wiley-Scrivener, [2020] 9781119614227 (DLC) 2019050429

Nutraceuticals and human blood platelet function: applications in cardiovascular health

LCCN	2018000730
Type of material	Book
Personal name	Duttaroy, Asim K., author.
Main title	Nutraceuticals and human blood platelet function: applications in cardiovascular health / by Asim K. Duttaroy.

Edition	First edition.
Published/Produced	Hoboken, NJ: John Wiley& Sons Ltd, 2018.
Description	1 online resource.
ISBN	9781119376057 (epub)
	9781119376002 (pdf)
LC classification	RC672
Summary	"A comprehensive review of the impact of dietary nutraceuticals on platelet function and its relationship to cardiovascular disease"--Provided by publisher.
Contents	Human blood platelets and their role in the development of cardiovascular disease -- Epidemiology of cardiovascular disease -- N-2 fatty acids and human platelets -- Effects of garlic, onion, ginger and tumeric on platelet function -- Herbs and platelet function -- Tomato extract and human platelet function -- Dietary nitrates and their antiplatelet effects -- Kiwifruit and human platelet function -- Polyphenols and human platelets -- Effects of ginkgo biloba, ginseng green tea, and dark chocolate on human blood platelet function -- Plant alkaloids and platelet function -- Strawberries and human platelet function -- Effects of metal ions on platelet function -- Individual compounds isolated from plant sources with anti-platelet activity.
Subjects	Cardiovascular Diseases--prevention & control
	Cardiovascular Diseases--etiology
	Dietary Supplements
	Functional Food
	Platelet Activation--physiology
Notes	Includes bibliographical references and index.
	Description based on print version record and CIP data provided by publisher.
Additional formats	Print version: Duttaroy, Asim K., author. Nutraceuticals and human blood platelet function First edition. Hoboken, NJ: Wiley, 2018 9781119376019 (DLC) 2018000528

Nutraceuticals and human blood platelet function: applications in cardiovascular health

LCCN	2018000528
Type of material	Book
Personal name	Duttaroy, Asim K., author.
Main title	Nutraceuticals and human blood platelet function: applications in cardiovascular health / by Asim K. Duttaroy.
Edition	First edition.
Published/Produced	Hoboken, NJ: Wiley, 2018.
ISBN	9781119376019 (hardback)
LC classification	RC672
Summary	"A comprehensive review of the impact of dietary nutraceuticals on platelet function and its relationship to cardiovascular disease"--Provided by publisher.
Contents	Human blood platelets and their role in the development of cardiovascular disease -- Epidemiology of cardiovascular disease -- N-2 fatty acids and human platelets -- Effects of garlic, onion, ginger and tumeric on platelet function -- Herbs and platelet function -- Tomato extract and human platelet function -- Dietary nitrates and their antiplatelet effects -- Kiwifruit and human platelet function -- Polyphenols and human platelets -- Effects of ginkgo biloba, ginseng green tea, and dark chocolate on human blood platelet function -- Plant alkaloids and platelet function -- Strawberries and human platelet function -- Effects of metal ions on platelet function -- Individual compounds isolated from plant sources with anti-platelet activity.
Subjects	Cardiovascular Diseases--prevention & control Cardiovascular Diseases--etiology Dietary Supplements Functional Food Platelet Activation--physiology
Notes	Includes bibliographical references and index.
Additional formats	Online version: Duttaroy, Asim K., author. Nutraceuticals and human blood platelet function

First edition. Hoboken, NJ: Wiley, 2018 9781119376002 (DLC) 2018000730

Pain erasers: the complete natural medicine guide to safe, drug-free relief

LCCN	2021012413
Type of material	Book
Personal name	Cook, Michelle Schoffro, author.
Main title	Pain erasers: the complete natural medicine guide to safe, drug-free relief / Michelle Schoffro Cook, PhD, DNM.
Published/Produced	Dallas, TX: BenBella Books, Inc., [2021]
Projected pub date	2109
Description	1 online resource
ISBN	9781953295859 (ebook)
	(trade paperback)
LC classification	RB127
Summary	"Within these pages, Pain Erasers: A Natural Doctor's Guide to Safe, Drug-Free Relief will reveal new ways to naturally erase your pain, often permanently! You'll discover dozens of natural painkillers, from a little-known but highly effective resin from the rainforest, along with such standbys as ginger and turmeric. And to boost the effects of these remedies, you'll get helpful tips on how to change your diet and lifestyle for optimal health and pain and inflammation management"-- Provided by publisher.
Subjects	Chronic pain--Alternative treatment--Popular works.
	Chronic pain--Prevention--Popular works.
	Self-care, Health--Popular works.
Notes	Includes bibliographical references and index.
	Description based on print version record and CIP data provided by publisher; resource not viewed.
Additional formats	Print version: Cook, Michelle Schoffro. Pain erasers Dallas, TX: BenBella Books, Inc., [2021] 9781953295514 (DLC) 2021012412

Pain erasers: the complete natural medicine guide to safe, drug-free relief

LCCN	2021012412
Type of material	Book
Personal name	Cook, Michelle Schoffro, author.
Main title	Pain erasers: the complete natural medicine guide to safe, drug-free relief / Michelle Schoffro Cook, PhD, DNM.
Published/Produced	Dallas, TX: BenBella Books, Inc., [2021]
Description	x, 262 pages; 23 cm
ISBN	9781953295514 (trade paperback) (ebook)
LC classification	RB127 .C685 2021
Summary	"Within these pages, Pain Erasers: A Natural Doctor's Guide to Safe, Drug-Free Relief will reveal new ways to naturally erase your pain, often permanently! You'll discover dozens of natural painkillers, from a little-known but highly effective resin from the rainforest, along with such standbys as ginger and turmeric. And to boost the effects of these remedies, you'll get helpful tips on how to change your diet and lifestyle for optimal health and pain and inflammation management"-- Provided by publisher.
Subjects	Chronic pain--Alternative treatment--Popular works.
	Chronic pain--Prevention--Popular works.
	Self-care, Health--Popular works.
Notes	Includes bibliographical references and index.
Additional formats	Online version: Cook, Michelle Schoffro, Pain erasers Dallas, TX: BenBella Books, Inc., 2021. 9781953295859 (DLC) 2021012413

Plants for weight loss: myth and reality

LCCN	2020043026
Type of material	Book
Personal name	Sirotkin, Alexander V., author.
Main title	Plants for weight loss: myth and reality / Alexander V. Sirotkin.

Published/Produced	New York: Nova Science Publishers, [2020]
Description	x, 183 pages; 23 cm.
ISBN	9781536187007 (hardcover)
	(adobe pdf)
LC classification	RM222.2 .S5575 2020
Summary	"This is a unique book which critically summarizes the current scientific knowledge concerning manifestations, mechanisms, consequences and prevention of dysfunctions of metabolism of fat, as well as the main known functional food and medicinal plants which can be and which cannot be used for prevention and treatment of obesity. The provenance, biologically active molecules, positive and adverse side-effects on health, influence on obesity and potential applicability of tea, chicory, Garcinia cambogia, Hoodia gordonii, chia, Irvingia gabonensis, apple cider vinegar, coffee, konjac/glucomannan, flaxseed, mulberry, oat, sweet and hot peppers, carob, cinnamon, plum, Cissus quadrangularis, Stevia rebaudiana, Yacon and ginger are described in details. In addition, less-known plants and plant molecules, as well as their combinations considered applicable for obesity treatments, are listed. It is demonstrated that more than half of the plant-based anti-obesity products available on the market are not properly clinically tested, or such tests, when performed, provided negative results. In addition, the author provides the reader with some practical advices and tips to combat obesity with healthy lifestyle. This book combines deep scientific analysis of physiological processes and popular form of their description. Such form enables to use this knowledge and advices for scientists, doctors, producers, distributers and consumers of functional food and medicinal plants, as well as for the common readers interested in healthy nutrition and life style"-- Provided by publisher.
Subjects	Reducing diets.

	Medicinal plants.
	Functional foods.
Additional formats	Online version: Sirotkin, Alexander V., Plants for weight loss - New York: Nova Science Publishers, 2021. 9781536187472 (DLC) 2020043027
Series	Nutrition and diet research progress

Plants for weight loss: myth and reality

LCCN	2020043027
Type of material	Book
Personal name	Sirotkin, Alexander V., author.
Main title	Plants for weight loss: myth and reality / Alexander V. Sirotkin.
Published/Produced	New York: Nova Science Publishers, [2021]
Description	1 online resource
ISBN	9781536187472 (adobe pdf)
	(hardcover)
LC classification	RM222.2
Summary	"This is a unique book which critically summarizes the current scientific knowledge concerning manifestations, mechanisms, consequences and prevention of dysfunctions of metabolism of fat, as well as the main known functional food and medicinal plants which can be and which cannot be used for prevention and treatment of obesity. The provenance, biologically active molecules, positive and adverse side-effects on health, influence on obesity and potential applicability of tea, chicory, Garcinia cambogia, Hoodia gordonii, chia, Irvingia gabonensis, apple cider vinegar, coffee, konjac/glucomannan, flaxseed, mulberry, oat, sweet and hot peppers, carob, cinnamon, plum, Cissus quadrangularis, Stevia rebaudiana, Yacon and ginger are described in details. In addition, less-known plants and plant molecules, as well as their combinations considered applicable for obesity treatments, are listed. It is demonstrated that more than half of the plant-based anti-obesity products available on the market are not properly clinically

tested, or such tests, when performed, provided negative results. In addition, the author provides the reader with some practical advices and tips to combat obesity with healthy lifestyle. This book combines deep scientific analysis of physiological processes and popular form of their description. Such form enables to use this knowledge and advices for scientists, doctors, producers, distributers and consumers of functional food and medicinal plants, as well as for the common readers interested in healthy nutrition and life style"--Provided by publisher.

Subjects	Reducing diets.
	Medicinal plants.
	Functional foods.
Notes	Includes bibliographical references and index.
	Description based on print version record and CIP data provided by publisher; resource not viewed.
Additional formats	Print version: Sirotkin, Alexander V.. Plants for weight loss New York: Nova Science Publishers, [2021] 9781536187007 (DLC) 2020043026
Series	Nutrition and diet research progress

Sustained energy for enhanced human functions and activity

LCCN	2017297285
Type of material	Book
Main title	Sustained energy for enhanced human functions and activity / edited by Debasis Bagchi.
Published/Produced	London: Elsevier/Academic Press, [2017]
Description	xxviii, 514 pages: illustrations; 25 cm
ISBN	9780128054130 (hbk)
	0128054131 (hbk)
LC classification	QP141 .S86 2017
Related names	Bagchi, Debasis, 1954- editor.
Summary	Sustained Energy for Enhanced Human Functions and Activity addresses the basic mechanistic aspects of energy metabolisms, the chemistry, biochemistry and pharmacology of a variety of botanical ingredients, micronutrients, antioxidants, amino

Contents acids, selected complexes, and other nutracueticals which have demonstrated a boost in and the sustainability of functional energy. The role of exercise and physical activity is also discussed, and the conclusion addresses paradigm shifts in the field and envisions the future.Intended for researchers and industry professionals, the book is as an essential reference on the impact of proper nutrient balance on sustained energy.-- Source other than the Library of Congress

Information theory and the thermodynamic efficiency of biological sorting systems / Chérif F. Matta, Lou Massa -- Roles of AMP, ADP, ATP, and AMPK in healthy energy boosting and prolonged life span / Durgavati Yadav, Yamini B. Tripathi, Prabhakar Singh, Rajesh K. Kesharwani, Raj K. Keservani -- An overview of nitrite and nitrate / Nathan S. Bryan -- An overview on nitric oxide and energy metabolism / Safia Habib, Moinuddin, Asif Ali -- Antioxidants and mitochondrial bioenergetics / Sushil Sharma -- Protein, carbohydrates, and fats / Prabhakar Singh, Rajesh K. Kesharwani, Raj K. Keservani -- Role of selected medicinal plants in sports nutrition and energy homeostasis / Marijana Zovko Končić -- Withania somnifera / Muzamil Ahmad, Nawab J. Dar -- An overview on Tribulus terrestris in sports nutrition and energy regulation / Andrzej Pokrywka, Barbara Morawin, Jaroslaw Krzywański, Agnieszka Zembroń-Lacny -- The use of Maca (Lepidium meyenii) for health care / Myeong Soo Lee, Tae-Hun Kim, Hye Won Lee -- An overview on Rhodiola rosea in cardiovascular health, mood alleviation, and energy metabolism / Michael Duncan, Neil D. Clarke -- Energy and health benefits of shilajit / Sidney J. Stohs, Kanhaiya Singh, Amitava Das, Sashwati Roy, Chandan K. Sen -- An overview on ginseng an energy metabolism / Haojun Zhang, Dongliang Wang, Wenwen Ru, Yufeng Qin, Xiangshan Zhou -- Glycyrrhiza glabra (licorice) / Wang Xiaoying, Zhang Han, Wang Yu -- An overview of yohimbine in sports medicine / Nevio Cimolai -- Black ginger extract enhances physical fitness performance and mususcular endurance / Kazuya Toda, Hiroshi Shimoda -- Role of marine nutraceuticals in cardiovascular health / Se-Kwon Kim, Isuru Wijesekara -- Royal jelly in medicinal to functional energy drinks / Hiroyoshi Moriyama, Manashi Bagchi, Debasis Bagchi -- Role of caffiene in sports nutrition / Lucas Guimarães-Ferreira, Eric T. Trexler, Daniel A. Jaffe, Jason M. Cholewa -- Beneficial roles of caffiene in sports nutrition and beverage formulations / Dawn E. Anderson -- Amino acids and energy metabolism / Kohsuke Hayamizu -- Branched chain amino acids and sports nutrition and energy homeostasis / José Miguel Martinez Sanz, Aurora Norte, Ella Salinas Garcia, Isabel Sospedra -- HMB supplementation / Fernanda Lima-Soares, Christian E.T. Cabido, Kassiana Arújo Pessôa, jason m. Cholewa, Carlos E. Neves Amorim, Nelo E. Zanchi -- Antioxidants and vitamins / Prabhakar Singh, Rajesh K. Kersharwani, Raj K. Keservani -- Salient features for designing a functional beverage formulation to boost energy / Anand Swaroop, Manashi Bagchi, Hiroyoshi Moriyama, Debasis Bagchi -- Caffiene-containing energy drinks/shots / Bill J. Gurley, Rick Kingston, Sheila L. Thomas -- An overview on the constituents and safety of energy / John P. Higgins, Karan Bhatti -- Interactions of commonly used prescription drugs with food and beverages / Sheila M. Wicks, Temitope O. Lawal, Nishikant A. Raut, Gail B. Mahady.

Subjects   Nutrition.
Functional foods.
Vitality.
Energy Metabolism.
Functional Food.
Dietary Supplements.

	Nutritional Physiological Phenomena.
	Exercise--physiology.
	Health & Fitness / Healthy Living.
	Health & Fitness / Holism.
	Health & Fitness / Reference.
	Medical / Preventive Medicine.
	Functional foods.
	Nutrition.
	Vitality.
Notes	Includes bibliographical references and index.

The "I love my instant pot" anti-inflammatory diet recipe book: from orange ginger salmon to apple crisp, 175 easy and delicious recipes that reduce inflammation

LCCN	2019023101
Type of material	Book
Personal name	Flaherty, Maryea, author.
Main title	The "I love my instant pot" anti-inflammatory diet recipe book: from orange ginger salmon to apple crisp, 175 easy and delicious recipes that reduce inflammation / Maryea Flaherty of HappyHealthyMama.com, author of Anti-inflammatory drinks of health.
Published/Produced	New York: Adams Media, [2019]
Description	223 pages: color illustrations; 23 cm
ISBN	9781507210994 (trade paperback)
	(ebook)
LC classification	TX840.P7 F55 2019
Summary	"Chronic inflammation is a major health risk and can wreak havoc on your body, contributing to many types of diseases. But preventing and/or reducing inflammation doesn't have to be an overwhelming challenge. Diet-particularly one high in processed, fatty, and sugary foods-is one of the main causes of chronic inflammation, but by introducing anti-inflammatory meals into your diet, you can reduce inflammation and enjoy a healthier lifestyle. The Instant Pot can be used to create healthy anti-inflammatory meals that are quick, easy, and most

	importantly delicious. With 175 recipes and photographs throughout, this cookbook is perfect for those who follow an anti-inflammatory diet. Whether you are new to the Instant Pot or an expert, this easy-to-understand cookbook takes you step-by-step through exactly how the Instant Pot works and offers simple recipes that anyone can follow. The "I Love My Instant Pot®" Anti-Inflammatory Diet Recipe Book shows you how to make satisfying, whole-food dishes from breakfast to dinner and from snacks to dessert. Discover how quick and easy it is to follow the anti-inflammatory diet using everyone's favorite cooking appliance. This cookbook makes creating healthy recipes in your Instant Pot easier than ever!"-- Provided by publisher.
Subjects	Pressure cooking. One-dish meals. Quick and easy cooking. Cooking. Cookbooks.
Form/Genre	Cookbooks.
Notes	"Authorized by Instant Pot." Includes index.
Series	"I love my" series

The all-day fat-burning cookbook: turbocharge your metabolism with more than 125 fast and delicious fat-burning meals

LCCN	2016053798
Type of material	Book
Personal name	Elkaim, Yuri, 1980- author.
Main title	The all-day fat-burning cookbook: turbocharge your metabolism with more than 125 fast and delicious fat-burning meals / Yuri Elkaim.
Published/Produced	New York, NY: Rodale, [2016]
Description	xiii, 242 pages: color illustrations; 24 cm
ISBN	9781623366070 (hardback: acid free paper)
LC classification	RM222.2 .E43317 2016

	Bibliography
Summary	" New York Times bestselling author Yuri Elkaim provides the perfect companion to The All-Day Fat-Burning Diet, arming you with quick and easy recipes following the 5-Day Food Cycling Formula. The All-Day Fat-Burning Cookbook includes more than 125 delicious gluten-, dairy-, and soy-free recipes including 5-minute, 5-ingredient refined sugar-free Coconut Cream with Berries; delicious 15-minute Beef and Rice with Spice; vegetarian BBQ Butternut Squash Steaks; and 3-minute, refined sugar-free Spicy Ginger Ale. These satisfying recipes are laid out according to the revolutionary 5-Day Food Cycling plan outlined in The All-Day Fat-Burning Diet and act as the perfect guide to help you stay lean and happy for life. "-- Provided by publisher. "Lose that stubborn weight while enjoying delicious food with this perfect companion to The All-Day Fat-Burning Diet. In The All-Day Fat-Burning Diet, renowned fitness expert and New York Times bestselling author Yuri Elkaim revealed the innovative way to reset and accelerate metabolism to burn fat 24/7. You were introduced to the 5-day food-cycling method, which helps supercharge metabolic rate while significantly improving health. Now, The All-Day Fat-Burning Cookbook makes following the plan a breeze, with quick-and-easy recipes that are presented according to the 5-day food-cycling formula. You will enjoy more than 125 delicious gluten-, dairy-, and soy-free recipes, including 5-minute, 5-ingredient Whipped Coconut Cream and Berries; flavorful, 15-minute Beef and Rice with Spice; and vegetarian BBQ Butternut Squash Steaks. These satisfying recipes will help you stay lean and happy for life"-- Provided by publisher.
Contents	All-day fat-burning principles -- How to make healthy eating stick for life -- Preparing your fat-burning kitchen -- Breakfasts -- Smoothies -- Sides

	-- Dips, snacks, and toppings -- Salads -- Bowls and quick-fix lunches -- Soups -- Mains -- Desserts -- The 10-day metabolic reset.
Subjects	Reducing diets--Recipes.
	Weight loss--Recipes.
	Fat--Metabolism.
	Cooking / Health & Healing / Weight Control.
	Health & Fitness / Weight Loss.
Form/Genre	Cookbooks.
Notes	Includes bibliographical references and index.
Additional formats	Online version: Elkaim, Yuri, 1980- author. All-day fat-burning cookbook Emmaus, Pennsylvania: Rodale, [2017] 9781623366087 (DLC) 2016056927

The cookie cure: a mother/daughter memoir of cookies and cancer

LCCN	2017030949
Type of material	Book
Personal name	Stachler, Susan, author.
Main title	The cookie cure: a mother/daughter memoir of cookies and cancer / Susan and Laura Stachler.
Published/Produced	Naperville, Illinois: Sourcebooks, [2018]
ISBN	9781492637837
LC classification	RC265.6.S73 A3 2018
Related names	Stachler, Laura, author.
Summary	"When twenty-two-year-old Susan Stachler was diagnosed with cancer, her mother, Laura, was struck by déjà vu--the same illness that took her sister's life was now attacking her daughter. Heartbroken but steadfast, Laura pledged to help Susan through the worst of her treatments. When they discovered that Laura's homemade ginger cookies soothed the side effects of Susan's chemo, both mother and daughter were inspired to start a business. Now, with Susansnaps, the duo sells their cancer-fighting cookies across the country. Told with admirable grace and infinite hope, The Cookie Cure is about more than baked goods and cancer-- it's about fighting for your life and for your dreams."-- Provided by publisher.

Subjects	Stachler, Susan--Health.
	Cancer--Patients--United States--Biography.
	Businesswomen--United States--Biography.
	Cookie industry--United States.
	Mothers and daughters--United States.
Dewey class no.	362.19699/40092 B

The covid chronicles: lessons from New Zealand

LCCN	2020445510
Type of material	Book
Personal name	Little, Paul, 1957- author.
Main title	The covid chronicles: lessons from New Zealand / Paul Little.
Published/Produced	Auckland, New Zealand: HarperCollinsPublishers, 2020.
	©2020
Description	289 pages; 24 cm
ISBN	9781775541691 (paperback)
	(ebook)
LC classification	RA644.C67 L58 2020
Summary	"For the first time in history, on 15 March 2020 the New Zealand government closed the country's borders. What followed was a story unprecedented in almost every way imaginable. ...The Covid Chronicles is a multi-stranded account of one of the most extraordinary times in Aotearoa's history, and the lessons we must heed for our future"--Back cover.
Subjects	COVID-19 (Disease)--Government policy--New Zealand.
	COVID-19 (Disease)--New Zealand--Anecdotes.
	COVID-19 (Disease)--Economic aspects--New Zealand.
	COVID-19 (Disease)--New Zealand--Psychological aspects.
	COVID-19 (Disease)--Political aspects--New Zealand.
	COVID-19 (Disease)--Social aspects--New Zealand.

Bibliography 129

Notes	New Zealand--History--21st century. Featuring: Jim Boult (Queenstown Lakes District mayor), Rohan Cahill-Fleury (primary school teacher), Jenene Crossan (CEO and co-founder, Flossie), Chris Farrelly (City Missioner, Auckland City Mission), Professor Juliet Gerrard (Prime Minister's Chief Science Advisor), Sam Hardy (mental health advocate), Sam Johnson (chief executive and founder Student Volunteer Army), Roger King (co-director Hakanoa Handmade, makers of ginger beer and syrups), Sido Kitchin (magazine editor), Helen McCarthy (producer Kerre McIvor Mornings, Newstalk ZB), Bill Newson (E tū union), Deborah Pead (founder of We Are Pead), Chris Quin (CEO Foodstuffs North Island), Michelle Sarich (co-principal Te Kura Kaupapa Māori o Hokianga), Mark Stewart (accountant), Francis and Kairora Tipene (funeral directors), Gary and Vicki Wallace (real estate salespeople), Mark Wallbank (restaurateur), Dr Siouxsie Wiles, MNZM (microbiologist and Associate Professor at the University of Auckland), and Mark Wilson (senior public relations and media officer, Mental Health Foundation).
Additional formats	Online version: COVID chronicles 9781775492009

The everything metabolism diet cookbook

LCCN	2015024458
Type of material	Book
Personal name	Boyers, Lindsay.
Main title	The everything metabolism diet cookbook / Lindsay Boyers, CHNC.
Published/Produced	Avon, Massachusetts: Adams Media, [2016]
Description	304 pages; 24 cm.
ISBN	9781440592287 (paperback) 1440592284 (paperback)
LC classification	RM222.2 .B64826 2016

130   Bibliography

Summary	"A cookbook of recipes intended for those looking to best utilize and cater to their metabolism"--Provided by publisher.
Subjects	Reducing diets--Recipes.
	Weight loss--Endocrine aspects.
	Metabolism--Regulation.
	Health & Fitness / Diets.
Notes	"Includes veggie-packed scrambled eggs, spicy lentil wraps, lemon spinach artichoke dip, stuffed filet mignon, ginger mango sorbet, and hundreds more!"--Cover.
	Includes index.
Series	An Everything series book

The fully raw diet: 21 days to better health with meal and exercise plans, tips, and 75 recipes

LCCN	2015037776
Type of material	Book
Personal name	Carrillo-Bucaram, Kristina, author.
Main title	The fully raw diet: 21 days to better health with meal and exercise plans, tips, and 75 recipes / Kristina Carrillo-Bucaram.
Published/Produced	Boston: Houghton Mifflin Harcourt, 2016.
Description	271 pages: color illustrations; 23 cm
ISBN	9780544559110 (paperback)
LC classification	RM236 .C29 2016
Summary	"The must-have book for FullyRaw fans or anyone who wants to explore a raw-foods vegan diet to lose weight, gain energy, and improve overall health and wellness The Fully Raw Diet offers a 21-day plan to help people enjoy a clean, plant-based, healthful approach to eating. Kristina Carrillo-Bucaram transformed her own health by eating vegetables, fruits, nuts, and seeds--100% fresh, raw, and ripe--and she is now the vivacious, uber-healthy founder of the FullyRaw brand. Her ten-year success with this lifestyle inspires thousands via social media, and her 21-day FullyRaw Video Challenge on YouTube in 2014 dramatically grew her fan base.

	This book shares her advice and will correspond to a new video challenge, with meal and exercise tips, recipes, and vivid photos. Fans will love the smoothies, salads, main dishes, and desserts, such as Lemon-Ginger Blast, Spicy Mango Basil Salad, Yellow Squash Fettuccine Alfredo, Melon Pops, and Caramel-Apple Cups"-- Provided by publisher.
Subjects	Raw food diet.
	Vegetarianism.
	Cooking (Vegetables)
	Raw foods--Therapeutic use.
	Cooking / Vegetarian & Vegan.
	Cooking / Health & Healing / Weight Control.
Form/Genre	Cookbooks.
Notes	Includes index.

The ginger and turmeric companion: natural recipes and remedies for everyday health

LCCN	2019037334
Type of material	Book
Personal name	Scherr, Suzy, author.
Main title	The ginger and turmeric companion: natural recipes and remedies for everyday health / Suzy Scherr.
Published/Produced	New York, NY: The Countryman Press, a division of W. W. Norton & Company Independent Publishers Since 1923, [2019]
ISBN	9781682683767 (paperback)
	(epub)
LC classification	TX819.G53 S34 2019
Summary	"More than 75 ways to support health and wellness with ginger and turmeric Likely already sitting on your spice rack, ginger and turmeric have been culinary and medicinal staples for centuries-and for good reason. While best known for their flavor, and turmeric's vibrant color, these spices are also rich in health benefits. Packed with vitamins, minerals, and antioxidants, ginger stimulates digestion, strengthens immunity, and helps ease motion sickness, while turmeric can help relieve migraines

	and even spice up your makeup regimen. Both have powerful anti-inflammatory properties. In The Ginger & Turmeric Companion, Suzy Scherr demonstrates how to incorporate these natural wellness aids into daily life. From surprising and delicious recipes-including information on how to maximize the benefits of adding ginger and turmeric to your diet-to health and beauty secrets, she presents a fuss-free guide to these powerful spices. With Scherr's comprehensive guidance, look no further than the spice cabinet for a feel-good, look-good way to mix up everyday routines"-- Provided by publisher.
Subjects	Ginger.
	Cooking (Ginger)
	Cooking (Turmeric)
Form/Genre	Cookbooks.
Notes	Includes index.
Series	Countryman pantry

The Korean kimchi cookbook: 78 fiery recipes for Korea's legendary pickled and fermented vegetables

LCCN	2017050959
Type of material	Book
Personal name	Kim, Man-jo, 1928- author.
Uniform title	Kimchʻi chʻŏnnyŏn ŭi mat. English
Main title	The Korean kimchi cookbook: 78 fiery recipes for Korea's legendary pickled and fermented vegetables / by Kim Man-Jo, Lee O-Young, Lee Kyou-Tae.
Published/Produced	Tokyo: Tuttle Publishing, [2018]
Description	120 pages: color illustrations; 22 x 27 cm
ISBN	9780804848602 (paperback)
LC classification	TX806 .K5613 2018
Related names	Yi, Ŏ-ryŏng, 1934- author.
	Yi, Kyu-tʻae, 1933- author.
Summary	"Kimchi is the newest star on the Asian culinary stage. These kimchi recipes are an appetizing way to add more vegetables with probiotics, vitamins, and enzymes to your health-conscious diet. This

	delicious Korean superfood is tasty in a surprisingly tangy, spicy, and pungent way! The Korean Kimchi Cookbook is the first Korean food cookbook in English to present Korean kimchi recipes in so many different forms -- and to fully explain the alchemy of fermentation and its health benefits, which include healthy digestion, anti-aging results, lowered cholesterol, and a stronger immune system. The Korean Kimchi Cookbook features the extensive history and background information about Korea's cuisine and fascinating culture. There are 82 flavorful and easy to prepare recipes organized by season including: Fresh Oyster Kimchi Swiss Chard Kimchi Fresh Ginger Pickles Traditional Cabbage Kimchi"-- Provided by publisher.
Subjects	Kimchi.
	Cooking, Korean.
	Cooking / Methods / Canning & Preserving.
	Cooking / Regional & Ethnic / Asian.
Form/Genre	Cookbooks.
Notes	Includes index.

The rainbow juice cleanse: lose weight, boost energy, and supercharge your health

LCCN	2014951438
Type of material	Book
Personal name	Southall, Ginger, author.
Main title	The rainbow juice cleanse: lose weight, boost energy, and supercharge your health / Dr. Ginger Southall.
Published/Produced	Philadelphia: Running Press, [2015] ©2015
Description	192 pages: illustrations; 21 cm
Links	Publisher description https://www.loc.gov/catdir/enhancements/fy1622/2014951438-d.html
	Contributor biographical information https://www.loc.gov/catdir/enhancements/fy1702/2014951438-b.html
ISBN	9780762457342 (hardcover)

	0762457341 (hardcover)
LC classification	RM255 .S68 2015
Summary	Offers a detox and weight-loss program using fruit and vegetable juices from every color of the rainbow, including rhubarb gingerade, minty pepper orange juice, and purple sea asparagus.
Subjects	Vegetable juices--Therapeutic use.
	Vegetable juices.
	Fruit juices--Therapeutic use.
	Fruit juices.
	Detoxification (Health)
	Reducing diets--Recipes.
Notes	Includes bibliographical references and index.

The whole30: the 30-day guide to total health and food freedom

LCCN	2015007139
Type of material	Book
Personal name	Urban, Melissa.
Main title	The whole30: the 30-day guide to total health and food freedom / Melissa Hartwig and Dallas Hartwig; with Chef Richard Bradford; photography by Alexandra Grablewski.
Published/Produced	Boston: Houghton Mifflin Harcourt, 2015.
Description	ix, 421 pages: color illustrations; 24 cm
ISBN	9780544609716 (hardcover)
LC classification	RA784 .H373 2015
Variant title	Whole thirty
	Whole 30
Related names	Hartwig, Dallas.
	Grablewski, Alexandra, photographer.
Summary	"Millions of people visit Whole30.com every month and share their stories of weight loss and lifestyle makeovers. Hundreds of thousands of them have read It Starts With Food, which explains the science behind the program. At last, The Whole30 provides the step-by-step, recipe-by-recipe guidebook that will allow millions of people to experience the transformation of their entire life in just one month. Melissa and Dallas Hartwig's critically-acclaimed

Whole30 program has helped hundreds of thousands of people transform how they think about their food, bodies, and lives. Their approach leads to effortless weight loss and better health--along with stunning improvements in sleep quality, energy levels, mood, and self-esteem. Their first book, the New York Times best-selling It Starts With Food, explained the science behind their life-changing program. Now they bring you The Whole30, a stand-alone, step-by-step plan to break unhealthy habits, reduce cravings, improve digestion, and strengthen your immune system. The Whole30 features more than 100 chef-developed recipes, like Chimichurri Beef Kabobs and Halibut with Citrus Ginger Glaze, designed to build your confidence in the kitchen and inspire your taste buds. The book also includes real-life success stories, community resources, and an extensive FAQ to give you the support you need on your journey to "food freedom.""-- Provided by publisher.

Subjects   Diet therapy--Popular works.
Nutrition--Popular works.
Food habits--Popular works.
Self-care, Health--Popular works.
Weight loss--Popular works.
Health & Fitness / Weight Loss.
Health & Fitness / Nutrition.
Cooking / Health & Healing / General.
Cooking / Health & Healing / Weight Control.

Notes   Includes index.

Your fit pregnancy: nutrition & exercise handbook

LCCN   2015452932
Type of material   Book
Personal name   Willick, Erica, author.
Main title   Your fit pregnancy: nutrition & exercise handbook / Erica Willick.
Published/Produced   New York: Sterling, [2016]
©2016

Description	ix, 278 pages, 8 unnumbered pages of plates: illustrations (some color); 23 cm
Links	Contributor biographical information https://www.loc.gov/catdir/enhancements/fy1703/2015452932-b.html Publisher description https://www.loc.gov/catdir/enhancements/fy1703/2015452932-d.html
ISBN	9781454916932 (paperback) 1454916931 (paperback)
LC classification	RG558.7 .W55 2016
Summary	"Positive and accessible, Your Fit Pregnancy breaks down exercise and nutrition into a trimester-by-trimester guide, with workouts (focusing on strength training, cardio, and yoga and stretching), plus meal plans and 50 recipes like Pumpkin Granola Yogurt Parfait, Smoky Corn and Edamame Beef Chili, and Simple Ginger Soy Poached Salmon. Author Erica Willick is a mother, two-time North American fitness champion, and founder of Sisters in Shape who also write a blog about pre- and postnatal fitness and health. She says in the introduction, '...these principles and programs were made to help you navigate through your pregnancy journey healthier and even fitter,'"-- Page [4] of cover.
Contents	Your Fit and Healthy Pregnancy -- Your Fit First Trimester -- Core Confidence and Pelvic Floor Power -- Your Fit Second Trimester -- Your Fit Third Trimester -- Your Fit Post-Baby: Building to Last -- Preggo Power Recipes -- Your Fit Pregnancy Exercise.
Subjects	Exercise for pregnant women. Physical fitness for pregnant women. Pregnancy--Nutritional aspects. Exercise for pregnant women. Physical fitness for pregnant women. Pregnancy--Nutritional aspects.
Notes	"Trimester-By-Trimester"--Cover. Includes bibliographical references (pages 272-273) and index.

Index

A

access, 41, 92, 93
accessibility, 92, 93
accommodation, 12
acetone, 8
acid, 2, 9, 10, 16, 22, 24, 30, 72, 99, 125
active compound, 57
active oxygen, 17
additives, 81
adhesion, 30, 60
adipose tissue, 62
adolescents, 12
ADP, 122
adsorption, 31
adults, 31
adverse effects, 8, 9
Africa, 1, 75, 77
age, 7, 25, 41
ageing population, 59
agonist, 28
alkaloids, 20, 115, 116
allergy, 15
alternative medicine, vii, 16, 19, 34
alternative treatments, 6
amino acids, 122, 123
amylase, 58
anaerobic bacteria, 24
analgesic, 28
anemia, 66
angiogenesis, 25
anti-asthma, 102, 104
antibacterial activity, viii, 19, 20, 22, 23, 29, 30, 32, 33, 34
antibiotic, 65
anti cancer, 25
anticoagulant, 26
anti-inflammatory, viii, 9, 13, 19, 20, 22, 26, 55, 57, 59, 60, 62, 65, 70, 71, 74, 76, 124, 132
anti-inflammatory medications, viii, 19, 22
antioxidant, vii, 4, 10, 15, 19, 22, 23, 26, 33, 58, 59, 61, 74, 76, 86, 87, 102, 105, 106
antipyretic, 28
anxiety, 7, 72
anxiety disorder, 72
apex, 45
aphthous ulcers, 28
apoptosis, viii, 24, 56, 60, 61, 62
appetite, 26
ARC, 14
arthritis, 2, 57, 59, 62
Asia, viii, 1, 55, 56
Asian countries, 99
asparagus, 102, 104, 134
assessment, 15, 33, 72
asthma, viii, 2, 55, 57
athletes, 4
atmospheric pressure, 39
ATP, 122
aversion, 12
avian influenza, 35
avoidance, 8

B

background information, 133
bacteria, 23, 28, 30, 33, 34, 35, 89
bacterial pathogens, 28
bacterium, 10, 35
beef, 100
beer, 98, 100, 129

beneficial effect, vii, viii, 4, 6, 7, 8, 11, 56, 58
benefits, vii, viii, 2, 23, 26, 34, 55, 57, 65, 66, 68, 69, 70, 71, 82, 84, 85, 86, 87, 98, 99, 122, 131, 133
benign, 28
beverages, 4, 42, 85, 98, 123
bile, 57
bioavailability, 2, 3
biochemistry, 121
biological activities, 20, 59
biosynthesis, 6, 16, 28, 83, 84
bitters, 97
bleeding, 26
blood, 3, 7, 16, 26, 58, 62, 114, 115, 116
body weight, 3
bone, 100
boosters, 101, 103, 104, 105
bowel, 6, 16
brain, 6, 68, 74, 76
Brazil, 55
breakdown, 22
bronchitis, 26
bronchodilator, 26
budding, 78
burn, 126

C

caffeine, 106
calcium, 5, 31, 66
calorie, 94
CAM, 13
canals, 29, 34
cancer, viii, 2, 4, 10, 25, 26, 56, 57, 60, 61, 65, 70, 71, 90, 91, 127
cancer cells, 25, 65
cancer therapy, 26
candidiasis, 27
carbohydrates, 22, 58, 122
carbon atoms, 2
carbon tetrachloride, 23, 74, 76
carcinogen, 10
cardiovascular disease, 115, 116
Caribbean, 82, 83
caries, 21, 30, 35
carob, 119, 120
carotenoids, 61

case study, vii, viii, 37, 42, 43, 45, 46, 48
Catharanthus roseus, 75, 77
cation, 28
cellulose, 53
central nervous system, 5, 8
Chad, 79
challenges, 88
chemical, 2, 11, 16, 29, 31, 33, 51
chemical characteristics, 33
chemicals, 23, 102, 105
chemokines, 22
chemoreceptors, 5
chemotherapeutic agent, 8, 20, 26
chemotherapy, 8, 17, 60
chicken, 100
children, 7, 12, 15, 29, 31
China, viii, 20, 39, 49, 55, 57
cholesterol, viii, 2, 56, 57, 95, 96, 133
chromatography, 23, 61
chronic diseases, 58, 59
chronic renal failure, 26
cigarette smoking, 72
classification, 56, 65, 66, 67, 69, 70, 72, 74, 76, 78, 79, 81, 82, 83, 84, 85, 87, 88, 89, 90, 92, 93, 95, 96, 97, 99, 100, 101, 103, 106, 107, 108, 111, 115, 116, 117, 118, 119, 120, 121, 124, 125, 127, 128, 129, 130, 131, 132, 134, 136
cleaning, 29, 67, 68, 80
climate, 47
clinical trials, 5, 12, 32, 61, 78
cocoa, 53
coconut oil, 52, 66, 67, 68
coffee, 69, 106, 119, 120
colic, 88
collagen, 65
colon cancer, 26, 60
colonization, 28
color, 68, 70, 77, 81, 82, 85, 88, 90, 93, 100, 107, 124, 125, 130, 131, 132, 134, 136
colorectal cancer, 61
communication, 24
community, 135
complement, 69, 88
complexity, 39
complications, 10, 58, 61, 62, 75, 77

Index

composition, vii, viii, 20, 33, 38, 39, 40, 43, 99
compounds, viii, 2, 3, 38, 39, 55, 57, 59, 60, 61, 62, 74, 75, 76, 77, 115, 116
conduction, 45
conductivity, 47
conference, 54
Congress, 66, 68, 107, 122
conservation, 101, 102, 104, 105
constipation, 8, 17, 88
constituents, 2, 3, 4, 5, 13, 17, 20, 31, 38, 62, 103, 105, 123
consumers, 119, 121
consumption, vii, viii, 1, 4, 7, 55, 56, 57, 87, 102, 103, 104, 105
control group, 58
controlled trials, 62
controversial, 8
cooking, 39, 83, 89, 94, 99, 125
cooling, 41
correlation, 48
cosmetic, 45
cost, 16, 41, 56
cough, 26, 38
Council of Europe, 49
COX-2 enzyme, 28
creativity, 97
crop, vii, 19, 20, 83, 85, 102, 105
cryopreservation, 101, 102, 104, 105
CTA, 13
cultivars, 58, 63
cultivation, 56, 57
culture, 82, 99, 133
curcumin, 2, 9
cure, 29, 95, 96, 127
cuticle, 45
cycling, 126
cyclooxygenase, 22, 59
cytokines, 22, 59
cytotoxicity, 61

D

danger, 26
debridement, 29
decay, 21
dehydration, 2, 5
delayed gastric emptying, 10
dental care, 109, 112
dental caries, 20, 30
dentin, 30
dentist, 108, 112
dentures, 33
Department of Agriculture, 63
deposits, 27
depression, 7
deprivation, 80
depth, 41
derivatives, 60, 61
diabetes, 2, 26, 34, 58, 61, 62, 63, 70, 71, 75, 76, 77, 83, 85
diabetic patients, 10
diarrhea, 3, 4, 26
dielectric constant, 40
diet, 60, 67, 70, 72, 74, 76, 79, 80, 88, 94, 99, 107, 117, 118, 120, 121, 124, 129, 130, 131, 132
digestion, 4, 20, 57, 62, 80, 90, 131, 133, 135
dipoles, 39
directors, 129
discomfort, 4, 7, 28
disease prevention, 56, 90, 91
diseases, vii, viii, 1, 4, 11, 16, 20, 30, 34, 55, 57, 58, 124
disorder, 27, 28
displacement, 41
dissatisfaction, 6
distillation, 38
distress, 3
distribution, 39, 41
diuretic, 102, 104
diversity, 2
DNA, 10
doctors, 95, 96, 119, 121
dogs, 8, 16
dosage, 83, 85
drug discovery, 102, 104
drug release, 25
drug resistance, 27
drug therapy, 75, 77, 111, 114
drugs, 6, 8, 15, 20, 31, 60, 109, 112
drying, 38, 39, 43, 61
dyslipidemia, vii, 19
dyspepsia, 4, 7, 12, 13

E

editors, 74, 76, 77

education, 69
electric field, 39, 40
electrical conductivity, 40
electromagnetic, 39
electron microscopy, 42, 44
emotion, 5
enamel, 31, 35
endangered, 102, 105
endothelial cells, 25
endotoxins, 30
endurance, 123
energy, 39, 40, 46, 48, 70, 71, 121, 122, 130, 133, 135
environment, 42, 108, 111
enzymes, viii, 4, 10, 15, 22, 23, 25, 56, 57, 59, 63, 75, 77, 132
epidermis, 45
epithelium, 28
equipment, 40, 42
erosion, 10
esophagus, 4
ethanol, 9, 15, 22, 26
ethyl acetate, 30
etiology, 115, 116
everyday life, 65, 69
evidence, 2, 8, 11, 12, 48
exercise, 4, 72, 122, 130, 131, 135, 136
extraction, vii, viii, 37, 38, 39, 40, 41, 42, 43, 44, 45, 46, 47, 48, 52
extraction technologies, 38
extraction yield, viii, 37, 43, 46, 48
extracts, 10, 12, 16, 22, 25, 27, 29, 30, 33, 34, 35, 52, 58, 59, 60, 61, 74, 76, 83, 84

F

fasting, 26
fat, 94, 119, 120, 125, 126, 127
fatty acids, 115, 116
FDA, 3
feces, 3
female rat, 3
fermentation, 133
fetal development, 17
fetus, 6
fever, 102, 104
fibers, 22
fitness, 126, 136
flavonoids, 20, 23

flavor, viii, 38, 55, 56, 68, 94, 97, 131
flour, 2
flowers, 97, 100
folklore, 102, 104
food, viii, 2, 3, 11, 12, 15, 20, 39, 42, 53, 55, 57, 80, 81, 88, 90, 91, 94, 98, 99, 106, 119, 121, 123, 125, 126, 131, 133, 134, 135
food additives, 2
Food and Drug Administration, vii, 3, 19, 32
food intake, 3
food products, 2
formation, 23, 27
formula, 126
free radicals, 9, 10, 59
freedom, 134, 135
friction, 39
fruits, 85, 86, 97, 130
functional food, 99, 119, 120
fungal infection, 27, 33

G

gallstones, 95, 96
gamma radiation, 15, 25
gastric mucosa, 17
gastric ulcer, vii, 1, 4, 9
gastroenteritis, 4
gastrointestinal disorders, v, vii, 1, 2, 3, 4, 11, 12, 13, 19
gastrointestinal tract, vii, 1, 4, 14
gene expression, 74, 76
genes, 22, 24
genus, 62, 74, 76
geographical origin, 38, 43
Germany, 108
ginger oil, 9, 14, 20, 22, 30, 31, 38, 43, 45, 46, 47, 48, 50
gingival, 20, 28
gingivitis, 28, 33, 34
ginseng, 8, 99, 102, 105, 115, 116, 122
GIS, 3, 8
gland, 44, 45
glasses, 106
glucagon, 7
glucose, 26, 58, 62, 83, 85
glucose tolerance, 58
GLUT4, 26, 63
glutathione, 10, 25

Index 141

glycolysis, 23
glycoproteins, 78
GRAS, vii, 3, 19
Greeks, 56
growth, 3, 10, 14, 16, 60
growth factor, 14
growth rate, 60
guidance, 132
guidelines, 15

H

hair loss, 65
half-life, 3
halitosis, 31
happiness, 100
hardness, 30
harmful effects, 11
harvesting, 2
headache, viii, 55, 57
healing, 56, 69, 91, 100, 107
health care, 62, 73, 95, 96, 102, 104, 108, 112, 122
health care system, 73
health effects, vii, 1
health information, 73
health promotion, vii, viii, 56, 57, 60
heart disease, 70, 71
heartburn, 3, 68
heat transfer, 45
heavy metals, 61
Helicobacter pylori (H. pylori), vii, 1, 10, 14, 16
hemoglobin, 26
hepatotoxicity, 26
herbal medicine, 4
herpes labialis, 31
herpes simplex, 35
herpes simplex virus type 1, 35
hexane, 22
history, 14, 69, 95, 97, 99, 128, 133
homeostasis, viii, 56, 57, 58, 83, 85, 122
hormones, 7, 60
horses, 107
host, 31
human, 3, 8, 9, 10, 14, 17, 45, 48, 74, 75, 76, 107, 114, 115, 116, 121
human health, 48, 74, 75, 76, 107
human subjects, 17

hybrid, 52
hydrocarbons, 21, 38
hydrogenation, 2
hydrophobicity, 23
hydroxyl, 23
hyperemesis gravidarum, 12
hyperglycemia, 10, 13, 101, 104
hyperlipidemia, viii, 55, 57
hypersensitivity, 7
hypertension, 75, 77, 103, 105
hypotensive, 102, 104

I

ibuprofen, 29
identification, 20
ileum, 4
image, vii, viii, 37, 38, 42, 43, 44, 48, 102, 103, 104, 105
image processing of the extract, viii, 37, 38
immune response, 23
immune system, 133, 135
immunity, 101, 103, 104, 105, 131
improvements, 135
in vitro, vii, 1, 4, 11, 16, 34, 35, 63
in vivo, 11
incidence, 30, 58, 59, 60
India, viii, 1, 19, 20, 38, 55, 56, 57, 68, 84, 85, 102, 105
Indians, 38
individuals, 20
induction, viii, 10, 48, 56
induction time, 48
industries, 42, 45, 48, 59, 103, 105, 108, 112, 122, 128
infection, vii, 1, 31, 34, 68
inflammation, 2, 10, 13, 23, 28, 62, 63, 68, 70, 71, 101, 102, 104, 117, 118, 124
inflammatory disease, 59
information technology, 73
ingredients, 2, 21, 32, 66, 68, 79, 80, 82, 91, 94, 95, 97, 98, 99, 107, 121
inhibition, viii, 15, 20, 28, 35, 56, 58, 59, 60, 62, 75, 77
inhibitor, 6
injury, 17, 74, 76
innate immune response, 78
insulin, viii, 26, 56, 58

insulin resistance, viii, 56, 58
integrity, 24, 31
intelligence, 95, 97
intervention, 72
intravenously, 3
ions, 31, 39
iron, 88
irradiation, 39, 45
irrigation, 29
irritable bowel syndrome, vii, 1, 7, 12, 16
Islam, 13, 15, 34, 61
Israel, 13, 51
issues, 26, 90, 101, 104

J

Japan, 106
joint pain, 67
joints, 95, 96
Jordan, 93

K

K^+, 16
ketones, vii, 19, 32
kidneys, 58
Korea, 132, 133

L

Lactobacillus, 30
landscape, 73
latency, 8
LDL, 57, 59
lead, 5, 6, 58, 80, 90
learning, 98
lens, 44
lesions, 9, 27, 31, 35
life quality, vii, 1
lifestyle changes, 90
lifetime, 80
lipid peroxidation, 4, 10, 15, 17, 23, 25, 59
lipids, 62
liposomes, 26
liquids, 25, 42
lithium, 12
liver, 3, 14, 15, 16, 58, 61, 74, 76
liver cancer, 61

localization, 45
love, 81, 124, 125, 131
lower esophageal sphincter, 7, 14
lymphoma, 62

M

magnitude, 40
Malaysia, 37, 49, 51
management, 26, 31, 33, 72, 75, 76, 101, 102, 104, 108, 117, 118
marketing, 102, 103, 104, 105
mass, 23, 39, 61, 88
mass spectrometry, 23, 61
materials, 39, 40, 42
matrix, 39, 40
matter, 38
Mauritius, 50, 51
measurements, 9
meat, 67, 68, 79
media, 129, 130
median, 7
medical, 42
medication, 25, 26, 72
medicine, vii, viii, 2, 6, 12, 19, 32, 42, 55, 69, 70, 95, 96, 97, 99, 102, 104, 107, 117, 118, 123
Mediterranean, 56
mellitus, 58, 61, 62, 75, 76
menopause, 95, 96
mental health, 90, 129
mental illness, 72
meta-analysis, 12, 61, 62
metabolic disorders, 62
metabolism, 3, 16, 58, 59, 67, 68, 119, 120, 122, 125, 126, 129, 130
metabolites, 3, 17, 38
metabolized, 3
metal ions, 115, 116
methanol, 30
methodology, 38, 43, 52
mice, 4, 14
micronutrients, 121
microorganisms, 3, 21, 29
microsomes, 15
microwave assisted-hydrodistillation, 38, 39, 40, 41, 46, 47
microwave heating, 40
microwave radiation, 63
microwaves, 39, 47

Index

Middle East, 56
migraines, 131
Ministry of Education, 49
models, 59, 72
modifications, 42
molecules, 4, 20, 39, 45, 119, 120
monoterpenoids, 38, 43
morbidity, 4
morphogenesis, 78
mortality, 3, 4
motion sickness, 6, 8, 26, 131
mucin, 26
multiple factors, 7
multiplication, 31
musculoskeletal, vii, 19

N

nanoparticles, 26
natural compound, 60
natural food, 98
natural products, 1, ii, 20, 38, 50, 108, 109, 112
Natural Resources Conservation Service, 63
nausea, vii, 1, 2, 5, 6, 7, 8, 9, 11, 12, 13, 14, 15, 16, 17, 20, 26
negative effects, 22
Nepal, 20
networking, 35
neural system, 58
neurohormonal, 4
New Zealand, 51, 86, 128, 129
Nigeria, 32, 47
nitrates, 115, 116
nitric oxide, 59, 122
nitric oxide synthase, 59
nitrite, 122
nitrogen, 4
nodules, 60
non-steroidal anti-inflammatory drugs (NSAIDs), 9, 22
North America, 14, 88, 136
nutraceutical, 33
nutrients, 3, 70, 79, 81, 85, 88, 90, 91, 106, 122
nutrition, 25, 90, 99, 119, 121, 122, 135, 136

O

obesity, 58, 62, 101, 103, 104, 105, 119, 120
oil, 9, 10, 14, 20, 22, 23, 25, 30, 31, 32, 33, 38, 39, 40, 42, 43, 45, 46, 47, 48, 57, 83, 84, 99
oil production, 48
olive oil, 95, 96
operating costs, 48
operations, 84, 85
oral application, vii, viii, 20, 21, 27
oral cavity, 24, 27, 28, 30, 31, 34
oral diseases, viii, 20, 26, 32, 108, 112
oral health, 21, 108, 111
organism, 24
organs, 3, 45
oxidation, 59
oxidative stress, 24, 26, 58, 62, 74, 76

P

pain, 6, 7, 12, 28, 29, 34, 70, 71, 117, 118
palate, 88
paradigm shift, 122
parallel, 48
parasympathetic activity, 29
parenting, 88
parents, 15
pathogenesis, 4, 17, 77, 78
pathogens, 20, 23, 28, 30, 34, 83, 85
pathophysiology, 12
pathways, 10, 13, 22, 24, 62, 78
peptic ulcer, 10
peptide, 7
periodontal, 20, 24, 28, 33, 34
periodontal disease, 20, 24
periodontitis, 28
perseverance, 23
pests, 83, 85
pharmaceutical, 14, 45, 59, 102, 104
pharmacology, 13, 83, 84, 121
phenolic compounds, 21
Philadelphia, 133
photographs, 125
physical activity, 122
physical fitness, 123
physiology, 79, 115, 116, 124
phytomedicine, 34

phytosterols, 2
placebo, 6, 7, 10, 17, 33
plant processing, viii, 37, 38
plants, 20, 35, 42, 48, 61, 63, 74, 75, 76, 77, 101, 102, 103, 104, 105, 109, 112, 119, 120, 121, 122
plaque, 29, 34
platelet aggregation, 6, 16
platelets, 115, 116
polar, 3, 39
polarity, 39
policy, 92, 93, 128
polyphenols, 62
polysaccharide, 23
population, 11
pregnancy, 2, 5, 6, 11, 12, 13, 14, 15, 16, 17, 135, 136
preparation, 16, 43
prescription drugs, 123
preservation, 102, 105
preservative, 81
preventative care, 108, 111
prevention, vii, 1, 12, 20, 22, 28, 30, 56, 90, 91, 111, 114, 115, 116, 119, 120
primary school, 129
principles, 15, 33, 126, 136
probe, 41
probiotics, 132
producers, 119, 121
professionals, 122
pro-inflammatory, 59
proliferation, viii, 23, 25, 28, 56, 60, 61
prophylactic, 35
prophylaxis, 30
prostaglandins, viii, 9, 10, 13, 19, 22, 28
protection, viii, 19, 23, 56
proteolytic enzyme, 4
psychological stress, 7
public health, 58
pylorus, 9

Q

quality of life, 7, 8, 12
quercetin, 59
questionnaire, 4

R

radiation, viii, 13, 14, 19, 23, 60
radicals, 23
radio, 25, 47
radiotherapy, 8, 25, 29, 34
rainforest, 117, 118
Ramadan, 35, 59, 62
reactions, 3
reactive oxygen, 4
reactivity, 7
real estate, 129
reality, 118, 120
receptors, 6, 8, 15, 26, 28, 29, 58
recommendations, 9
recovery, 46, 90
recreational, 4
recurrence, 90, 92
regulations, 99
relief, 6, 65, 117, 118
remission, 91, 92
repair, 65
replication, 78
researchers, 6, 38, 45, 48, 102, 104, 122
residue, 43
resistance, 20
resolution, 44
resources, 135
response, 7, 8, 10, 22, 39, 52, 59
rhabdoviruses, 78
rheumatoid arthritis, viii, 55, 57, 59
rhizome, viii, 1, 24, 28, 33, 38, 43, 55, 56, 57, 61
risk, 5, 58, 61, 70, 71, 91, 92, 124
RNA, 78
rodents, 3
root canal treatment, 29
roots, 12, 25, 27, 29, 33, 34, 74, 76, 98
rotations, 39
routes, 25
routines, 132
rules, 99

S

saccharin, 8
safety, 2, 11, 12, 15, 17, 41, 56, 123
saliva, 29
salmon, 100, 124
salts, 57

Index

SARS, 26, 34
SARS-CoV, 26
scanning electron microscopy, 42, 44, 45
school, 7
science, 72, 75, 77, 103, 106, 134
scientific knowledge, 119, 120
scope, vii, viii, 20
SCT, 13
secretion, 9, 26, 29, 45, 57
security, 73
seed, 31, 38
self-esteem, 135
SEM model, 44
sensation, 28, 90
sensing, 24, 72
sensitivity, 30, 31, 58, 61
sensitization, 15
sensors, 41
serotonin, 58
serum, 3, 58, 61
services, 92, 93
sex steroid, 6
shade, 43
shape, 41
shrimp, 82
side effects, 4, 5, 7, 60, 127
signals, 5
signs, 29, 71
skin, 66, 67, 68, 69, 80
sodium, 30, 35
solvents, 52
Southeast Asia, vii
specialists, 108, 111
species, 4, 20, 30, 39, 45, 56, 61, 63
spice, vii, viii, 1, 11, 15, 42, 55, 56, 62, 63, 68, 126, 131
Sprague-Dawley rats, 17
spring, 82
standardization, 32
starvation, 5
state, vii, viii, 25, 37, 56
stimulation, 22, 59
stomach, 4, 26, 67
stomatitis, 28, 33, 78
storage, 45, 94
strength training, 136
stress, 15, 58, 67, 68, 90
stretching, 136
structure, 31, 44, 45, 46, 48, 78

styles, 58, 119, 121
substitutes, 25
sucrose, 23
sugarcane, 53
Sun, 13, 50
supplementation, 14, 58, 61, 123
supply chain, 102, 103, 104, 105
suppression, 24, 25, 28, 59
susceptibility, 34
sustainability, 122
sweeteners, 81
symptoms, 4, 5, 6, 7, 8, 12, 13, 95, 96
synthesis, viii, 6, 9, 19, 22, 23

T

tannins, 20, 23
taste aversion, 15
techniques, viii, 37, 42, 89
technologies, 13, 38, 72, 102, 105
teeth, 21, 34
temperature, 2, 38, 40, 42, 43, 45, 47, 48
terpenes, 2, 22, 57
testosterone, 6, 11
textbook, 108, 112
Thailand, 20
therapeutic effects, 21, 99
therapeutic use, 75, 77
therapeutics, ii, 102, 104
therapy, 2, 20, 26, 29, 61, 62, 71, 73, 90, 92, 99, 108, 111, 114, 135
thermal energy, 39
time use, 42
tissue, 28
tooth, vii, 19, 21, 23, 28, 29, 30
toxic effect, 3, 32, 60
toxicity, vii, 19, 23, 32, 33
toxicology, 16
trade, 70, 89, 102, 103, 104, 105, 117, 118, 124
transcription, 25, 78
transformation, 73, 134
treatment, vii, 1, 4, 5, 6, 7, 12, 15, 16, 17, 20, 26, 27, 28, 30, 32, 35, 45, 59, 60, 75, 77, 91, 117, 118, 119, 120
trial, 7, 15, 16, 17, 33, 34, 35
triggers, 91
tumor, viii, 24, 55, 57, 60

tumor cells, 60
tumor development, 25
Turkey, 1, 49
type 2 diabetes, 58, 61, 62

U

ulcer, 10, 17, 23, 28
uniform, 42
United Kingdom, 86, 96, 97
United States (USA) 63,66, 67, 77, 101, 103, 105, 128
universal access, 73
universities, 101, 104
upper respiratory tract, 26
USDA, 56

V

vaccine, 78
variations, 79
vascular endothelial growth factor, 24
vascular system, 16, 45
vegetables, 97, 130, 132
velocity, 7
virus infection, 35
virus replication, 78
vitamin B6, 5
vitamins, vii, 19, 22, 57, 123, 131, 132
volatility, 38
vomiting, vii, 1, 5, 6, 8, 9, 11, 12, 13, 14, 15, 16, 17, 26

W

war, 95, 96
Washington, 82
waste, 3
water, 39, 40, 41, 43, 45, 46
weight control, 72
weight loss, viii, 56, 58, 71, 90, 118, 120, 121, 134
well-being, 107
wellness, 68, 130, 131
West Indies, 1
Western countries, 99
worldwide, vii, viii, 11, 19, 42, 55, 56, 108, 112
wound healing, 28

X

xerostomia, 29, 34

Y

yield, viii, 37, 40, 43, 46, 47, 48

Z

Zingiber officinale, v, vii, viii, 1, 11, 12, 13, 14, 15, 16, 53, 55, 56, 57, 61, 62, 63, 83, 84
Zingiberaceae, viii, 1, 50, 55, 56